Sample	Methods	Analysis
random assignment	structured metric	differences between group means or sets of scores
nonrandom assignment to groups	structured	
stratified random or existing groups	structured	differences between group means or sets of scores
probability	structured	correlational analysis or tests of association
probability or total population	semistructured with some unstructured	descriptive statistics
theoretical or purposive sampling	unstructured qualitative	content analysis or constant comparison

Advanced Design in Nursing Research

Advanced Design in Nursing Research

EDITED BY

Pamela J. Brink
Marilynn J. Wood

SAGE PUBLICATIONS
The Publishers of Professional Social Science
Newbury Park   London   New Delhi

For information address:

SAGE Publications, Inc.
2111 West Hillcrest Drive
Newbury Park, California 91320

SAGE Publications Ltd.
28 Banner Street
London EC1Y 8QE
England

SAGE Publications India Pvt. Ltd.
M-32 Market
Greater Kailash I
New Delhi 110 048 India

Printed in the United States of America

Library of Congress Cataloging-in-Publication Data

Brink, Pamela J.
    Advanced design in nursing research / edited by Pamela J. Brink and Marilynn J. Wood.
        p.   cm.
    Bibliography: p.
    Includes indexes
    ISBN 0-8039-2742-8
    1. Nursing—Research—Methodology.   I. Wood, Marilynn J.
II. Title.
    [DNLM: 1. Nursing Research. 2. Research Design. WY 20.5 B858a]
RT81.5.B73   1989
610.73'072—dc20
DNLM/DLC
for Library of Congress   89-10096
                                                                  CIP

FIRST PRINTING 1989

Contents

Preface

In our first text, *Basic Steps in Planning Nursing Research: From Question to Proposal,* we organized the entire volume according to three levels of research based on knowledge of the topic. In order to help the beginner to plan research accurately, these levels of knowledge were presented throughout that text, from "how to ask a researchable question" to "how to write a research proposal." We acknowledge that these three levels of research could be further subdivided into many designs but believe the three-level approach is useful for the novice to learn the essential decision-making rules for planning research.

The current work follows that primary theme of three major designs based upon knowledge: exploratory-descriptive, survey, and experimental. In this book, however, we subdivide each of these three designs into two further levels and acknowledge that there are undoubtedly other levels as well, but those presented do cover the major designs utilized in nursing research and contribute an extremely useful way to classify research designs. Beginning with the experimental design, in which the researcher has the most control over the variables and their action, each subsequent design is contrasted with this model, and its strengths and weaknesses are viewed in relation to the classic or "true" experiment. Subsequent designs derive from the experimental design in logical order. The development of research and research designs has followed the basic concept of logical positivism found in Western philosophy, and this text follows the same tradition. Ordinal scales are known to be inexact, and this one is no exception. We do, therefore, provide other research approaches from nursing and other disciplines at the end of the text to explain how one uses and/or critiques designs that do not fit the presented model.

7

This text is offered to the advanced student or the teacher who used *Basic Steps in Planning Nursing Research* in their earlier days and found this schema useful but not sufficiently detailed to use as a graduate text and reference. We hope this text fills that need.

We would like to acknowledge the assistance of Gail Ardery, who critiqued our chapters for content and rhythm. Having used *Basic Steps*, she was thoroughly familiar with the Brink and Wood style of writing, thinking, and teaching nursing research. With her doctorate in linguistics, she was an invaluable asset to us. We would also like to thank the reviewers who critiqued the book, gave us invaluable advice, and encouraged us to go on. Finally, we thank the many students in Iowa and California who asked questions at each step along the way.

Pamela J. Brink
Marilynn J. Wood

PART I
INTRODUCTION

1. Introduction

Pamela J. Brink
Marilynn J. Wood

This text is based on the premise that theory and research are inextricably intertwined. Neither is useful in advancing nursing knowledge without the other. Theory provides explanations for why things happen the way they do. Research provides the means to test theory to determine whether its explanations hold true, and simultaneously leads to new ideas for theory construction. Accordingly, for research to be of value in the advancement of knowledge it must be closely and appropriately melded into the process of theory development. The basic principle put forth in this text is that the level of knowledge available on a research topic determines the level of design that can be used to study that topic. This principle cannot be overemphasized. Fawcett and Downs (1986), in *The Relationship of Theory and Research*, exemplify this principle by including in their appendices research reports representing the three basic levels of knowledge.

The function of this reader is to describe a number of research designs useful in nursing research. Each design is described using a standard format. The classical design is presented, along with its usual variations. One to three examples of the design, as they have appeared in the nursing literature, are provided. Strengths and weaknesses of each design in sampling, methods, reliability, validity, data analysis, and issues related to the use of human subjects are discussed. Finally, each chapter discusses issues that must be dealt with in relation to human subjects, proposal writing, and critiquing.

Two major concepts provide the basic organization of this text. The first is that research designs are based upon the level of knowledge (and therefore the level of theory) about the topic being studied. The second is that research designs can be categorized according to the degree of control each offers over the research situation. The designs in this book are ordered from the most highly controlled, or those in which a great amount of knowledge exists on the topic being researched, to the least controlled designs, or those for which little knowledge exists on the topic. *Control* refers to investigator regulation of the research variable(s). In other words, a *controlled* research variable is not allowed to interfere with the action of other variables. The investigator has sufficient knowledge about the actions and interactions of variables that they can be isolated and studied in precise ways, all of which are established by the investigator at the outset of a study. In other words, variables can be controlled during the data collection phase or the data analysis phase; but the decision as to when a variable will be controlled is made in advance of data collection. When a variable is controlled, it does not vary in any way other than the way the investigator has predetermined it to vary. When a variable varies by itself and the investigator only observes the variance and documents it, the situation or the variable is in control of the research situation, not the investigator.

TYPE OF RESEARCH DESIGN AND TERMINOLOGIES

Research studies may be described or classified in a variety of ways. Although all such classifications have their failings, taken together they provide a handy tool for identifying particular characteristics of each level of research. The following sets of terms, adapted from Nieswiadomy (1987) will be used throughout the text.[1]

Qualitative and Quantitative

The terms *qualitative* and *quantitative* refer both to the *method* of data collection and to the *type of data* collected. The distinguishing feature is whether the data to be collected are already enumerated, whether they can be collected and enumerated, or whether they must remain verbal descriptions. Data that are structured in the form of numbers or that can be immediately transposed into numbers are considered *quantitative*. Data that cannot be structured in the form of numbers are considered *qualitative*. Measurement—whether at the nominal, ordinal, interval, or ratio level—is the hallmark of quantitative designs. Quantitative methods attempt to measure phenomena on a numeric scale of some kind, producing data that reflect at least the *frequency* with which a phenomenon occurs, and at most an exact measure of the *amount* of the phenomenon occurring under prescribed circumstances. By nature, quantitative methods require substantial knowledge of the phenomena under study in order for tools to be available to measure these phenomena. In contrast, qualitative data collection methods are flexible and unstructured, capturing verbatim reports or observable characteristics, and yielding data that usually do not take a numerical form. Words, film, postcards, art, and all sensory data are considered qualitative data unless they are transformed into some numeric system. Qualitative data can serve as the bases for insights, grounded theories, categorizations, taxonomies, processes, or outcomes. (For further reading in qualitative nursing research, see Field & Morse, 1985; Leininger, 1985; Morse, 1988; Munhall & Oiler, 1986; Parse, Coyne, & Smith, 1985; Stern, 1980, 1985; Swanson & Chenitz, 1986; Wilson, 1985, 1986.)

The choice between qualitative and quantitative methods is based on the type of research design. Exploratory designs primarily use flexible, open-ended qualitative data collection methods, while descriptive designs combine qualitative and quantitative methods. All other designs may incorporate qualitative data collection as an enhancement to the data, but not as a primary data collection method. Although the qualitative-quantitative distinction is widely used to classify research, it provides only two vast categories, each containing numerous designs. We find it more useful to place designs on a continuum based on the amount of theory and knowledge each requires. By doing this, it becomes possible to envision a research program or a given topic moving along this continuum as knowledge and theory in that topic area evolve.

The Concept of Time in Relation to the Design

A number of design terms refer to the researcher's temporal perspective looking back in time or looking forward: retrospective, prospective, *ex post facto*, historical, longitudinal, and cross-sectional. *Retrospec-*

tive (or *ex post facto*) designs measure phenomena that have occurred earlier in time. Designs in which the outcome or dependent variable is known and the independent or causal variable is sought are correlational retrospective designs. All historical studies are also retrospective. *Prospective* designs, on the other hand, measure variables that will be occurring during the study. All experimental studies are prospective because they are based upon predictive hypotheses. Time-series designs are also prospective. *Longitudinal* is a term used, particularly by epidemiologists, to describe a prospective design that follows a cohort of subjects over time. The term *cross-sectional* describes designs conducted in the present time to examine what currently exists. The fundamental characteristics of cross-sectional designs is that all data are collected at one point in time. (See Polit & Hungler, 1987, for a more complete description of these concepts in relation to design.)

Location or Setting

Research may also be described according to location or setting, generally differentiating between *laboratory* and *field* studies.

Laboratory studies are conducted in controlled settings particularly suited to the experimental design. In addition to the traditional settings used by basic scientists, laboratory sites would include clinical research units within hospitals, rooms equipped with two-way mirrors or video equipment for studies of behavior, and facilities equipped with physiological monitoring equipment for studies of human physiological responses. In contrast, most observational nursing research is conducted in the "real" world or the "field." Although it is certainly possible to conduct a descriptive observational study in a laboratory setting, this is a more expensive method of conducting such a study and raises questions about the validity of the findings.

Field studies occur in natural settings, where people are behaving as they usually do. Data are collected in the field primarily by means of observation and questioning. Additional information is obtained through available data, photography, and so on. *Field settings* include not only Pacific islands and African villages, but hospital wards, classrooms, nursing homes, and clinics. Nurses do field research when they observe nurse-patient interactions in health care institutions, document student-teacher interactions in classrooms, or describe staffing patterns in hospitals. The type of setting chosen for a study depends on the research design. For example, an exploratory or descriptive study of the type and amount of foods people eat should be observed in a natural setting so that daily food choices, methods of preparation, and social setting for eating are as "usual" as possible. In contrast, a laboratory setting in which all foods are prepared and eaten under highly controlled circumstances would be useful if precise measurement of food intake were sought. Studies of the relationship between nutritional intake and weight reduction lend themselves nicely to highly controlled experiments conducted in clinical laboratory settings.

Applied Versus Pure Research

Another major distinction is made between "applied" and "pure" research. *Pure* research is undertaken for the sake of learning something new, of building knowledge, without concern for whether or not the knowledge can be utilized directly. Its purpose is simply to study the phenomenon, not to change human circumstances. The knowledge gained may or may not be directly usable and applicable to a present-day problem.

In contrast, the major purpose of *applied* research is to be directly usable and applicable to a current problem or issue. Applied research is undertaken to test whether some specified change can be effected and whether that change will be permanent (Foster, 1969). Searching for the causes of diseases such as cancer or AIDS is pure research. Testing interventions (or treatments) is *applied research*. Most nursing care research is applied. Any clinical experimental or comparative design that tests one nursing intervention technique against another is essentially an applied research study. Its purpose is to change something, to improve the human condition in some way, to improve the delivery of nursing care, or to alter some aspect of the patient environment. Not all experimental designs, however, are applied. Some experiments are conducted to increase knowledge only, to see what will happen in a controlled setting when variables are manipulated. Within a practice discipline such as nursing, however, most research will eventually be applicable to practice, although many different studies involving several levels of research may be required before application is possible.

Deductive Versus Inductive

Some texts use the terms *deductive* and *inductive* to designate whether research contributes to theory testing or theory building. The main thrust of theory testing is deductive. Experimental designs are by their very nature *deductive* or derived from theory. Their purpose is to test theory. Based upon data obtained in an experiment, an investigator either accepts or rejects a research hypothesis. Rejection entails "deducing" either that the theory was in error or that the experiment did not directly test the theory. Acceptance entails both deducing that the theory was correct and assuming that the experiment directly tested the theory. Deductive studies are usually empirical, more specific, fact based or "hard" data based, and not abstract.

Inductive studies, by contrast, are more abstract and general in scope, based upon "soft" data, less specific, usually using exploratory or descriptive designs and qualitative data collection methods for the purpose of building or creating theory. The process of deriving theory from an in-depth qualitative data collection project has been termed "grounded theory" (Glaser & Strauss, 1967; Hutchinson, 1986; Stern, 1980, 1985; Swanson & Chenitz, 1986; Wilson, 1986). These studies develop concepts from the data that are then used to develop theory. Inductive studies using phenomenological inquiry frequently result in a description of an experience. Correlational studies, although usually deductive, can also be inductive when significant relationships between variables lead to insight regarding cause and effect linkages. Descriptive designs can be either deductive or inductive.

Process Versus Content

Research endeavors may also be described as either process or content studies. Studies of grieving, dying, maturing, and crisis, for example, all examine a process, whereas studies of the incidence of disease, measurement of health attitudes, or the opinions of nurses regarding professional practice are content studies. The process-content distinction parallels the distinction between purely descriptive designs and purely exploratory designs. Most exploratory studies focus on process in an attempt to explain the phenomena under study. Descriptive studies, even longitudinal studies, describe phenomena or populations at a particular time period. Though descriptive data can be collected at several points in time, each data collection period constitutes a distinct cross-sectional study, as data are collected at one moment in time. Consequently, descriptive research findings neither describe a process nor explain how or why it works. Process studies frequently attempt to discover the stages people go through in response to a threat or particular stressor. For example, dying can be conceptualized as a process of moving from social life and living to social dying and eventual death. Bereavement has been studied as the process a person goes through in coping with death or other loss (Saunders, 1983). *Culture shock* (Brink & Saunders, 1976) is a term that refers to the process of adapting to a move from a familiar to an unfamiliar environment. The discovery of one's sexual identity has been considered a stressor to which the individual must adjust (Kus, 1985). Adjustment, of course, is a process. In process studies, therefore, the process is the content. Process studies examine how people adjust or adapt to change. Content studies in these areas might examine the numbers of persons failing to resolve the crisis encountered through the death of a significant other, comparisons of the adaption of men versus women to a move to an unfamiliar environment, or the numbers of persons in particular occupational groups who identify themselves as homosexual versus heterosexual. These cases simply examine a phenomenon as it exists either in different populations or within one population.

Experimental Versus Nonexperimental

Many texts label research studies as either experimental or nonexperimental. *Experimental* designs involve manipulation of the independent variable, whereas *nonexperimental* designs do not manipulate variables. This classification system is very limited, considering the enormous number of possible nonexperimental designs. In addition, this distinction is derived from, and tends to perpetuate, the belief that only experimental designs are "real" or "scientific" research.

THE DESIGN LABELS USED IN THIS BOOK

The design taxonomy used in this book is based upon the principle of control, or the degree to which the investigator is able to prevent any untoward variance among the variables under study. Control itself is based upon the current level of knowledge about the topic. The paradigm enumerated previously by Brink and Wood (1978, 1983, 1988) presents three basic levels of design—experimental, survey, and exploratory-descriptive—each of which contains two sublevels. These are carried forward into this book as follows:

- Level III: experimental designs
  - (a) experimental
  - (b) quasi-experimental
- Level II: survey designs
  - (a) comparative
  - (b) correlational
- Level I: exploratory-descriptive designs
  - (a) descriptive
  - (b) exploratory

Ideally, at successively higher levels of design, the degree of control and the level of knowledge about the variables increases. The level of knowledge about pertinent variables should be the greatest at the level of the experiment, and is expected to be most limited at the exploratory level.[2] Accordingly, the choice of an appropriate design is based upon the current level of knowledge (or theory) about the research topic. When a causal relationship among variables can be both predicted and ethically *tested*, experimental or quasi-experimental designs are warranted. If a researcher believes research variables are related and can predict the outcome of their interaction, but cannot ethically manipulate the independent variable, a comparative design may be used to test theory and safeguard living subjects at the same time. If the researcher has a basic descriptive knowledge about the individual research variables but does not know whether they are related, the design is best formulated at the correlational level. If, on the other hand, a variable or concept has been discovered through exploration but no information is available about its existence in particular populations, a descriptive design is appropriate. Finally, if very limited or no knowledge about the topic is available, an exploratory design is most appropriate. Control of variables and prediction of their action require extensive knowledge. If the outcome of an experiment cannot be predicted and supported with theory, it is unethical to conduct that experiment on living subjects.[3] Level of design is based, therefore, upon knowledge about the operations of the variables in the topic and the degree of control that can be exercised over these variables in the research process itself.

Theory is built and supported at each level of knowledge, so that when we speak of a knowledge base for research, we automatically assume a theory base. Since theory is built upon accepted knowledge to explain what is known, theory changes as knowledge changes. And because a careful building of facts is prerequisite to developing and testing theory, all levels of research design are needed to advance theory development in nursing. Moreover, theory building might require moving back and forth across the continuum of research designs, because acquiring knowledge might require returning to explore further topics once thought to be well understood.

Level III. The experimental level of research is designed to test theory in laboratory settings or in controlled clinical trials. The greater the degree of control in the research setting, the greater the confidence that the research findings are accurate.

The *experimental design,* the most highly controlled of all research designs, is amenable to laboratory study, entails manipulation of the independent variable(s), and requires control of all intervening variables. Based upon theory developed from previous research, each step in the experiment requires a predictive hypothesis regarding the effect of the independent on the dependent variable(s). All assumptions are spelled out and are either verified by previous research or tested by the current research. All logical steps between cause and effect are specified. The key issue for this design is *internal validity,* or the assumption that changes in the dependent variable are actually due to the independent variable. Experimental and control groups are created by random assignment. Ethical concerns for the protection of human and animal subjects are the most restrictive. Experimenters, more than any other kind of researchers, are required to establish that all subjects' rights are protected to the greatest degree possible and that potential harmful effects are counterbalanced by potential benefits. Data collection is quantitative and prospective. Data analysis is designed to discriminate between and among experimental and control groups. Although experimental studies are the most directly applicable to nursing practice because of their controlled samples, they are the least widely generalizable in and of themselves. This is simply due to the controlled narrowness of the study and sample. Experiments are designed to be repeated on many samples with small variations in the independent variable over time. A single experiment on a single small sample adds to the test of a part of the theory but not the entire theory. Many experiments with different samples may be required to increase generalizability to the point where findings can be widely applied in practice.

The *quasi-experimental design* is distinguished from the true experiment by the lack of random assignment of subjects to groups. This lack of control limits confidence in the internal validity of the study. Otherwise, the design is exactly the same as the experimental design. Data are predominantly quantitative, and data analysis distinguishes between and among treatments and among treatment groups. Many field experiments actually use a quasi-experimental design when the assignment of subjects to the various experimental and control groups cannot be controlled by the researcher.

Level II. At the survey level of research, prior research findings are available in the literature. These studies yield a statistical analysis of the relationships between and among variables.

The *comparative design* is used when a cause-and-effect relationship can be predicted between variables on the basis of previous research findings. This design subjects a theory to testing without manipulation of the independent variable. Comparative designs usually occur in field studies. The sample is selected on the basis of the presence or absence of the independent variable, thus creating comparative groups at the beginning of the study. There are times, however, when the groups are established during data analysis. Data are predominantly quantitative, and data analysis differentiates between and among groups. This design is used in both basic and applied research, often when the independent variable cannot be manipulated due to ethical constraints.

The *correlational design* examines the relationship between two or more variables when no previous research findings support a prediction of cause and effect. This design simply allows one to study the relationship of two or more variables based upon hunches or logical assumptions. The design is also appropriate when one is searching for possible causative variables or for a particular outcome variable. Although specific variables may be "assumed to be" independent or dependent on the basis of their temporal occurrence, their actual relationship can be determined only through correlational data analysis. Correlational designs are usually field studies rather than laboratory studies, basic rather than applied, cross-sectional rather than longitudinal, and either prospective or retrospective. They are based on quantitative data collection from large samples. Control is increased through reliability and validity testing of data collection instruments, sample selection procedures, and data analysis. The central issue in these studies is to establish generalizability or *external validity*.

Level I. At the *exploratory-descriptive level* of research, usually little or no theory or prior research has addressed the specific variable under study. Alternatively, prior research on the variable may have been conducted, but only in populations other than the one currently under study. The phenomena under study are either unknown or understudied, or, because of recent happenings, a reexploration is indicated. By utilizing flexible approaches to discovery, these studies attempt to provide either a total or "in the round" description of a variable, or an exploration of some process.

The *descriptive design* is used to describe a single variable or population completely, accurately, and thoroughly. Descriptive studies usually involve cross-sectional field research using both qualitative and quantitative data collection techniques. Examples include anthropological ethnographies and population surveys such as the U.S. Census. Data analysis includes a mixture of content analysis, taxonomies, and descriptive statistics. External validity is a major issue in descriptive studies of known populations that do not use the total available population. Because many descriptive studies are of unknown or understudied populations, representativeness is always an issue.

The *exploratory design* is the least controlled design. Its central purpose is to develop valid definitions of a concept, describe a process, or yield beginning theories that explain the phenomenon under study. Data are collected in depth and over time in order to increase the validity of the concept being developed. Consequently, samples are usually quite small (from one to twenty). Data are most frequently collected by means of a qualitative field study subjected to inductive analysis. Examples include phenomenological studies examining processes according to the perspective of the individuals undergoing the process, and the "grounded theory" or field study approach, using participant observation with intensive interviewing to observe and analyze a process as it occurs in order to explain why it occurs the way it does.

Other Types of Designs

Other types of designs presented in this book fit the control-based paradigm to varying degrees. They frequently represent examples of "mixed" designs, drawing upon elements of basic designs at multiple levels but not meeting all the criteria for any one level. They are presented separately because of their importance to nursing research.

Historical research is nonexperimental and is based upon available written data, artifacts, or oral histories, all of which are usually qualitative data. Historiography can be cross-sectional or longitudinal. Depending upon the question asked, the study may be comparative, correlational, descriptive, or purely exploratory. A critical step in historiography is establishing whether the data are primary or secondary, hearsay or eyewitness accounts, and true or falsified documents, and whether the data sources are biased or objective observers of the times. The process of data analysis involves a great deal of interpretation on the part of the researcher, and in this way is similar to the exploratory study. The variables under study, however, may be well known in the present day. The researcher has no control over the way in which the original data were collected, but a great deal of control over which data are included in the study and how these are interpreted. Although historical studies are just beginning to appear in the nursing research literature, their legitimacy is indisputable.

Like historical designs, *epidemiological* designs tend to mix elements of other designs, most frequently utilizing correlational designs but not limited to them. They can vary greatly in control over variables and level of knowledge. Their primary goal is to document health, illness, and disease patterns for the purpose of establishing prevention, intervention, or maintenance programs for health problems.

A third type of research given special attention in this text is the *methodological* study, used to develop and test data collection instruments. Although this area has been neglected in nursing research until recently, it is evolving into a specialty area. The methodological study can be part of a research project at any level, as its major purpose is to develop reliable and valid instruments. In instrument development, researchers often make use of all three levels of research, analyzing a concept at the exploratory level, and then developing and testing an instrument to measure this concept through the other levels. In the process, theory may be developed and tested as it relates to the concept. In this book, the major discussion of reliability and validity of measurement will be found in Chapter 12, on methodological research.

The fourth design type is the *evaluative* design. Many clinical and educational programs have attempted to change something in the current system, improve some practice, or enhance a problem-solving mechanism. All these programs need to be evaluated in some consistent fashion. Evaluative research is both descriptive, seeking to describe what has occurred, and experimental, testing the effect of some manipulation or change. Data can be either qualitative or quantitative, and usually both are included.

The last chapter is devoted to the *pilot study*. Frequently equated with exploration but rarely described in any detail, pilot studies are assumed to be the first step in any research plan and are sometimes published in the literature. The differentiation between exploratory designs as beginning stages of a planned program of research and pilot projects is critical.

This book has emerged as a result of our many years of looking for a good resource for graduate courses in advanced design. We hope that others will find this approach useful in helping them make decisions about the design of a research project.

NOTES

1. This classification of nursing research studies has been adapted from Nieswiadomy (1987, pp. 39-54).

2. We expect ethical researchers to have a great deal of knowledge about the effects on human subjects of the manipulation of the independent variable prior to inflicting the independent variable on them. For this reason, we state that knowledge at this level should be the highest, as we are intervening in people's lives. Although there may be an enormous knowledge base in survey designs, these designs are still descriptive, even when using complex statistical techniques.

3. One of the reasons there are such strict guidelines on the protection of human subjects in the United States today is that in the past many experiments were conducted on humans as "fishing expeditions"—to find out what would happen if this or that were manipulated. Some people died, some were harmed psychologically or physiologically for life, and babies were born deformed, among other results. These same studies would not be approved by institutional review boards today. Instead, all experiments on human and animal subjects must have some fact-based logical or theoretical outcomes predicted at the outset in order to be approved.

REFERENCES

Brink, P. J., & Saunders, J. M. (1976). Culture shock: Theoretical and applied. In P. Brink (Ed.), *Transcultural nursing: A book of readings*. Englewood Cliffs, NJ: Prentice-Hall.
Brink, P. J., & Wood, M. J. (1978). *Basic steps in planning nursing research: From question to proposal*. North Scituate, MA: Duxbury.

Brink, P. J., & Wood, M. J. (1983). *Basic steps in planning nursing research: From question to proposal* (2nd ed.). Monterey, CA: Wadsworth Health Sciences.

Brink, P. J. & Wood, M. J. (1988). *Basic steps in planning nursing research: From question to proposal* (3rd ed.). Boston: Jones & Bartlett.

Fawcett, J., & Downs, F. (1986). *The relationship of theory and research*. Norwalk, CT: Appleton-Century-Crofts.

Field, P., & Morse, J. (1985). *Nursing research: The application of qualitative approaches*. Rockville, MD: Aspen.

Foster, G. (1969). *Applied research*. Philadelphia: F. A. Davis.

Glaser, B., & Strauss, A. (1967). *The discovery of grounded theory*. Chicago: Aldine.

Hutchinson, S. (1986). Grounded theory: The method. In P. Munhall & C. Oiler (Eds.), *Nursing research: A qualitative perspective* (pp. 111-129). Norwalk, CT: Appleton-Century-Crofts.

Kus, R. (1985). Stages of coming out: An ethnographic approach. *Western Journal of Nursing Research, 7*(2), 177-193.

Leininger, M. (Ed.). (1985). *Qualitative research methods in nursing*. New York: Grune & Stratton.

Morse, J. (Ed.). (1988). *Qualitative nursing research: A contemporary dialogue*. Rockville, MD: Aspen.

Munhall, P., & Oiler, C. (Eds.). (1986). *Nursing research: A qualitative perspective*. Norwalk, CT: Appleton-Century-Crofts.

Nieswiadomy, R. M. (1987). *Foundations of nursing research*. Norwalk, CT: Appleton & Lange.

Parse, R., Coyne, A., & Smith, M. J. (1985). *Nursing research: Qualitative methods*. Bowie, MD: Brady.

Polit, D. F., & Hungler, B. P. (1987). *Nursing research*. Philadelphia: J. B. Lippincott.

Saunders, J. M. (1983). A study of widow bereavement involving various modes of death. In P. J. Brink & M. J. Wood, *Basic steps in planning nursing research: From question to proposal* (2nd ed., pp. 235-260). Monterey, CA: Wadsworth Health Sciences.

Stern, P. (1980). Grounded theory methodology: Its uses and processes. *Image, 12,* 20-23.

Stern, P. (1985). Using grounded theory method in nursing research. In M. Leininger (Ed.), *Qualitative research methods in nursing* (pp. 149-160). New York: Grune & Stratton.

Swanson, J. M., & Chenitz, W. C. (1986). *From practice to grounded theory: Qualitative research*. Menlo Park, CA: Addison-Wesley.

Wilson, H. S. (1985). *Research in nursing*. Menlo Park, CA: Addison-Wesley.

Wilson, H. S. (1986). Presencing: Doing grounded theory. In P. Munhall & C. Oiler (Eds.), *Nursing research: A qualitative perspective* (pp. 131-144). Norwalk, CT: Appleton-Century-Crofts.

Part II
EXPERIMENTAL DESIGNS

The primary purpose of experimental designs is to test theory. The significant difference between experimental designs and all other designs is that in experimental designs the independent variable is manipulated. The research question asks: What is the difference between groups after the independent variable has been altered and why does the alteration produce those differences? The question is answered with "Because . . ." and the explanation provides the theoretical framework for the study. These studies test one portion of a theory rather than the entirety of the theoretical position. Cause and effect is always predicted based upon theory. Predictive hypotheses are written at the beginning of the study, stating the precise nature of both the manipulation of the independent variable and its effect on the dependent variable. Manipulation of the independent variable tests theory in a manner not possible with any other design.

The two chapters in this section describe experimental and quasi-experimental designs. The single feature that distinguishes these two major designs from all other designs is the manipulation of the independent variable. No other designs have this feature. The true experiment provides the greatest control over the experimental situation: The experimental variable is manipulated, there is random assignment to groups, and there is at least one control group. *Internal validity* is the key issue in assessing the accuracy of the findings. Other critical features include control and the validity of the measure of the dependent variable. The quasi-experimental design, in contrast to the true experiment, lacks either a control group or random assignment to groups.

The classic work on experimental and quasi-experimental designs by Campbell and Stanley has been used by researchers in many disciplines since it was first published in 1963. Campbell and Stanley developed the concepts of *internal* and *external validity* as they apply to studies with human subjects in natural settings. In the two chapters that follow, Buckwalter and Maas have utilized this classic work, adapting the basic principles to make them relevant to nursing studies.

Because of the level of control and the strength of the theoretical base required to support an experimental or quasi-experimental design, these designs will be used as the basis for comparison for the other designs presented in this book.

2. True Experimental Designs

Kathleen C. Buckwalter
Meridean L. Maas

There are a number of strategies or research designs that can be employed in the systematic study of problems that are of interest to nurses. The experimental design is the appropriate research strategy when the questions to be answered require the testing of theory and causal relationships. Experiments, broadly defined, are tests that involve at least one treatment (independent variable), units (e.g., subjects) to be analyzed by assignment/nonassignment to a treatment, and a comparison for inferring effects that may be attributed to the treatment. Experimental designs are of two major types, true experiments and quasi-experiments, although in general persons use the term *experimental design* when referring to true experiments. In addition to the general characteristics listed above for experiments, *true experiments* include the random assignment of units to comparison groups for inferring a change that has been caused by a treatment. Random assignment is an essential component of true experiments that is designed to achieve comparability of comparison groups. *Quasi-experiments* have a treatment (independent variable), outcomes (dependent variable), and units to be analyzed; but random assignment of units is not included for determining the groups of units to be compared. True experiments are described in this chapter. Quasi-experiments are discussed in the following chapter. Throughout the remainder of this chapter, the terms *experimental design* and *true experiment* will be used interchangeably, unless otherwise noted.

AUTHORS' NOTE: *We wish to thank Joan Crowe and Nancy Goldsmith for typing the manuscript for this chapter.*

All experimental designs, true experiments, and quasi-experiments are appropriate for answering Level III questions (Brink & Wood, 1983), which seek to explain *why* a relationship exists, are proposed and answered within a theoretical context, and are theory testing in nature. The researcher who appropriately employs experimental designs begins from a position of logical relationships derived from current theory and research findings. All of these designs are powerful methods for testing hypotheses of causal relationships among variables. The emphasis is on four main criteria: (1) establishing causal relationships, (2) manipulating an independent variable, (3) measuring the impact of the independent variable on the dependent variable, and (4) minimizing or accounting for the effects of factors other than the independent variable on the dependent variable. However, the true experiment is the *most powerful* strategy for testing causal hypotheses and achieving the above four criteria, because random assignment is used to create the comparison between groups from which a change due to the treatment is inferred.

TYPES OF TRUE EXPERIMENTAL DESIGNS

There are a number of different experimental designs that meet the criteria for true experiments. These include the "classical" experimental design, the factorial design, the multiple treatment groups-repeated measures design, and the Solomon four-group design. While there are a number of additional variations on these designs, illustration of the use of these designs provides a basis for understanding the strengths and weaknesses of true experiments and for how variations can be structured to maximize strengths to study specific problems. An important assumption underlying all true experimental designs is that equivalence of groups is maintained throughout the course of the experiment and is not compromised by such things as differential attrition—that is, variable dropout rates that may make experimental and control subjects different on critical factors at the time of the analysis. If experimental and control groups become nonequivalent, the design then becomes quasi-experimental.

The "Classical" Experimental Design

All experimental designs are variations on the basic "classical" experimental design, which consists of two groups, an experimental and a control group, and two variables, an independent and a dependent variable. Units to be analyzed (e.g., subjects) are randomly assigned to each of the experimental and control groups. Units in the experimental group receive the independent variable (the treatment condition) that the investigator has manipulated. Subjects in the control group do not receive the independent variable treatment. The control group subjects are measured at the same time as the experimental group, although no planned change or manipulation has taken place with regard to the independent variable.

Factorial Designs

Classical experimental design allows the manipulation of a single variable at a time, holding all other conditions constant. Frequently, problems of interest to nurses are more complex than the classical design permits. Factors (variables) *interact* to produce behaviors of interest to nurse researchers. *Factorial designs* permit the manipulation of more than one independent variable at a time, and thus allow the simultaneous testing of multiple hypotheses. Further, interaction effects between variables are revealed, making factorial designs an important variation on the classical experimental design. Although the example used later in this chapter is a 2 × 2 factorial design, factorial experiments can be conducted with three or more independent variables (known as factors). Each factor must have two or more levels; thus when new factors are added, more hypotheses can be tested simultaneously. Concurrently, the interpretation of main effects and interaction effects becomes more complex with the addition of new factors. Factorial designs are also referred to as "levels of treatment" designs. When one of the factors cannot be manipulated, such as sex of subjects, it is referred to as a *blocking variable*, and the design that incorporates the blocking variable is known as the *randomized block design*.

Multiple Treatment Groups—Repeated Measures Design

This design uses several experimental groups, each of which receives a different treatment. Control is achieved through comparison among groups and from measures taken on the dependent variable for all groups at Time 1 and Time 2. It is not always true that a control group will be used that has no treatment at all. There can also be more than one pretest and posttest measure for the dependent variable for all groups.

Solomon Four-Group Design

This is a rigorous design for controlling effects on the dependent variable that may be due to factors other than the independent variable. However, it is used less often than other designs because a large group of homogeneous subjects is required to make up the four groups. It is difficult to introduce the treatment simultaneously for all groups in order to avoid extraneous temporal effects, and statistical analysis is complex. These problems will be clarified when they are discussed along with the research example later in the chapter.

Prior to the illustration of these four experimental designs with examples from the nursing research literature, the essential elements that characterize true experiments—their strengths and weaknesses, and issues of the research setting, measurement, and analysis—are described. This discussion will make the research examples more understandable and more useful.

ESSENTIAL CHARACTERISTICS OF EXPERIMENTAL DESIGNS

In experimental designs, the investigator predicts an experimental outcome based on theory and previous research findings to explain the results in the context of logical and tested relationships. Basically, the researcher hypothesizes that the dependent variable for the experimental group will be altered in some specific (predicted) way, whereas the same dependent variable for the control group will remain unchanged. In order to test a relationship and most confidently infer this result, experimental designs must be characterized by three essential elements: randomization, manipulation, and control.

Randomization

In a true experimental design, *randomization* refers to subjects being assigned by chance to either receive (the experimental group) or not receive (the control group) the treatment condition or intervention (independent variable). A number of procedures exist for assigning individuals to groups, such as a coin toss, random numbers table, or computerized random number generators. The key characteristic of all these procedures is that each subject has an *equal* and *known* probability of being assigned to either the control or the experimental group. If any subject has a greater or lesser chance of being assigned to either group, then the assignment process is not random, and the assumptions underlying a true experimental design are violated.

The advantage of assigning subjects to groups in a random manner is that this should result in the groups initially being similar to one another prior to the intervention. For example, imagine that a nursing intervention for treating depressed patients is being evaluated, and a group of persons who have been referred by their family physician to a community mental health center is used as subjects in the study. Half of these subjects are randomly assigned to participate in the treatment program, and the remaining subjects are placed on a waiting list as a control group. Based on this method of assigning participants to a condition, the two groups of depressed persons should not differ in their pretreatment level of depression or in other characteristics that may affect the treatment outcome (e.g., levels of social support). Assuming that the group receiving the nursing intervention is significantly less depressed than the control group following completion of the treatment program, then it becomes possible to conclude that the nursing intervention was responsible for the improvement in depression that occurred.

Random assignment to condition *does not guarantee* that the two groups will be similar to one another. Based on sampling theory, significant differences (at $p < .05$) between the two groups will occur in 1 out of 20 cases of assigning subjects to groups. Further, if the sample size is not large enough, significant variables may not be equally distributed among groups, even with random assignment. In this situation, the researcher may wish to consider some additional methods of distributing important variables, such as matching or use of a more homogeneous population (see also the discussion of control of extraneous variance, below). However, studies have consistently supported the efficacy of random assignment to condition over various ways of matching subjects who are participating in different groups (Sherwood, Morris, & Sherwood, 1975).

Manipulation

In experimental designs the causative variable must be amenable to manipulation by the investigator; that is, the researcher "does something" to subjects in the experimental condition. However, a word of caution is needed regarding the control group. Even though the researcher does not actively manipulate subjects in the control group, it is important that he or she be aware of what may be happening to them. Control groups should experience all the same things (including environmental factors and time spent with data collectors) as subjects in the experimental group, except, of course, the independent variable. Often, ethical considerations will prohibit manipulation of variables (e.g., introduction of pain or other aversive stimuli to subjects). Similarly, other variables cannot be manipulated (e.g., attitudes, age, disease, and other such attributional variables). Finally, organizational policy of the research setting may disallow manipulation of variables (such as making dietary changes or altering medication regimens). The ability of the researcher to manipulate the independent variable is a major source of control in experimental studies.

Control

Control is a key concept in experimental designs. Cook and Campbell (1979, p. 8) identify three uses of the term *control* in relation to research designs, all of which involve eliminating threats to valid inference. One type of control refers to the researcher's control over the research environment; a second refers to control over the experimental variable; and the third suggests the ability to identify and rule out threats to internal validity. This last type of control is typically achieved through the use of a comparison or control group and through attention to sources of variance. The control group consists of subjects whose scores on the dependent variable are compared to the scores of subjects who received the experimental condition. In experimental designs with more than one experimental group, control is present in the sense of a formal comparison between groups. In many nursing studies, control subjects receive the usual or traditional methods of care, rather than no treatment, against which the effects of the experimental intervention are measured.

A major strength of experimental designs is their ability to *control variance* or to take into account factors that may contribute to differences in the dependent variable. Three kinds of variance must be considered in order to provide valid answers to research questions: (1) systematic or experimental variance, (2) extraneous variance, and (3) error variance (Kerlinger, 1973, pp. 306-313).

Systematic or experimental variance refers to the systematic effect of the independent variable(s) on the dependent variable(s) and is a type of variance that should be *enhanced*. That is, experimental conditions should be planned to be as *unlike as possible*. Say an investigator wishes to determine the most effective way to teach psychiatric patients about their psychotropic medication regime by comparing the efficacy of a 1:1, nurse to individual patient, teaching program to that of a group teaching approach. To maximize systematic variance, the two teaching programs (experimental conditions) should be substantially different from each other so that the effects of teaching programs can be separated from the total variance of the dependent variable (in this case, patient knowledge of the medication regime), which is often largely due to chance.

Extraneous variance refers to the effects of extraneous variables (also referred to as "nuisance" or "unwanted" variables) on the dependent variable(s). This source of variance is to be *controlled* by the design, as extraneous variables are factors other than the independent variable that could lead to differences between groups. In addition to randomization, which is the most ideal way to control all possible extraneous variables simultaneously, Isaac and Michael (1971, p. 54) list four ways the researcher can control extraneous variance. All of these techniques require that the researcher know in advance which extraneous variables need to be controlled:

(1) *Building the extraneous variable into the design,* as an independent variable (e.g., if sex of subjects is considered an important variable in determining response to an intervention, a 2×2 factorial design with sex (male/female) as one of the factors, may be used).

(2) *Eliminating or holding constant* an extraneous variable by selecting subjects as homogeneous as possible on that variable (e.g., all elderly female subjects).

(3) *Matching* subjects on one or more extraneous variables, as long as those variables are highly correlated with the dependent variable(s) (e.g., matching subjects for rural/urban residency or type of disease). (Matching is *never* an adequate substitute for randomization and should be used only when other techniques are not feasible.)

( ) *Statistical* control of variance, such as analysis of covariance (ANCOVA).
This procedure is explained more fully in the section on data analysis.

Error variance refers to the variability of measures due to random fluc-
t ations, including errors of measurement. Control of error variance
i ; achieved in two main ways, by standardizing the measurement (ex-
)erimental) conditions, and by increasing the reliability of the measurement instruments.

(1) *Control of experimental conditions* can be enhanced by keeping factors such
as place, time of day, instructions to subjects, and experimental personnel constant. Otherwise, factors such as noise, hunger, fatigue, or anxiety may create errors of measurement.
(2) *The reliability of measurement instruments* (e.g., their accuracy) can be increased by writing items clearly, adding more similar items, and providing clear, consistent instructions (Kerlinger, 1973, p. 454). Unreliable
instruments increase error variance, and this in turn compromises the
effects of systematic variance.

Experimental designs are considered the most powerful research approach because they permit the researcher to maximize systematic
variance and to control for extraneous and error variance. This is principally a problem of establishing internal validity of the experiment.
Experiments, however, are often limited in generalizability because
they intrude on natural settings and subjects are not randomly selected
from a target population. They are powerful designs for controlling
threats to external validity, which are an important aspect of generalizability. Experimental designs are also the most powerful for testing
causal relationships.

Internal validity is the primary objective of experimental methodology.
The researcher essentially asks the question, ''Was the effect observed
on the dependent variable actually due to the action of the independent variable?'' Thus the nurse who is critiquing a proposal or published report using an experimental design will want to evaluate the
study in terms of how well it controls for extraneous variables that
might invalidate the results of the experiment by introducing rival and
plausible hypotheses. Cook and Campbell (1979) identified twelve types
of extraneous variables that, if left uncontrolled, may produce effects
that the researcher could mistake for the effect of the independent
variable. These threats to internal validity—history, maturation, testing,

instrumentation, statistical regression, selection, experimental mortality, selection/maturation interaction, diffusion or imitation of treatments, selection/history interaction, compensatory equalization of treatments, and compensatory rivalry by respondents receiving less desirable treatments—are explained briefly below and are discussed in relation to quasi-experimental designs in the next chapter.

- *History:* the events or circumstances other than the introduction of the treatment variable that occur coincident with the time interval between the pretest and posttest measurements.
- *Maturation:* changes within the subjects themselves that occur over time and that are not related to any specific event, such as tiring, gaining weight, or becoming more knowledgeable.
- *Testing:* the learning that results from being tested at Time 1 that affects responses to the test at Time 2, regardless of the introduction of the treatment variable.
- *Instrumentation:* changes that occur in the measurement instruments, observers, or raters that potentially produce changes in the dependent variable measurements.
- *Statistical regression:* the movement of mean scores from Time 1 to Time 2 that most often results when subjects are selected on the basis of scores that are at the extremes of the distribution.
- *Selection bias:* the selection of subjects on a nonrandom basis that may produce differences in the experimental and comparison group subjects with regard to the criterion measurement irrespective of the differential exposure to the treatment.
- *Experimental mortality:* nonequivalent attrition of subjects from the experimental and comparison groups.
- *Interactions with selection:* a number of the previously described threats to internal validity can interact with selection, causing spurious treatment effects. The combined effects of nonrandom selection of subjects and differential changes that occur within the subjects on dependent variable measurements between Time 1 and Time 2 may be interpreted as changes that are due to the treatment when in fact they result from selection and maturation interaction. Selection-history and selection-instrumentation are among the additional interaction effects that can be erroneously interpreted as treatment effects. Because of these types of interaction effects, subjects that are in any way self-selected should be scrutinized carefully for differential treatment effects at Time 2 even though the groups demonstrated equivalence on the dependent variable measurements at Time 1. Selection-maturation interaction occurs when some process within the subjects is changing at a differential rate regardless of the introduction of the treatment. Selection-history results when subjects are drawn from different

unique settings that have exposed the subjects to variable local historical events that may influence the outcome measure. Selection-instrumentation can result when subjects achieve different mean scores on an instrument that is not constructed with equal intervals, producing "ceiling" and "floor" effects on the measurement. When a ceiling effect occurs, a larger number of subjects in one group will be unable to achieve more true change in the measurement score. Conversely, when more subjects in one group are clustered at the lower end of a scale it may be because the instrument is not capable of measuring true scores below a certain point (floor effects).

- *Diffusion or imitation of treatments:* the introduction of a treatment that involves information when the experimental and control group subjects may be able to interact with one another, directly or indirectly, and learn about information intended for others. This threat to internal validity may be a particularly salient contaminating effect for many nursing research studies where subjects are physically proximal to one another and likely to communicate, as in a hospital ward area.

- *Compensatory equalization of treatments:* the use of an experimental treatment that has actual or potential value to subjects where authorities or subjects may be unwilling to tolerate an imposed inequity in the distribution of the treatment. The result may be that the treatment is obtained by subjects making up the control group so that the planned experimental contrast is compromised.

- *Compensatory rivalry by respondents receiving less desirable treatments:* the assignment of subjects to experimental and control groups where control group subjects are disadvantaged by the absence of the treatment in contrast to experimental subjects and thus are motivated to compete for equity. Like compensatory equalization, compensatory rivalry is a response to the inequity of benefits imposed by the presence of an experimental condition. However, compensatory equalization is mainly a response by administrators and compensatory rivalry is a response by subjects in a disadvantaged no-treatment group.

In general, experimenters are primarily concerned with the internal validity of their design. However, they are also interested in the *external validity*, or generalizability, of their findings with respect to other subjects, settings, and variables. The researcher and those critiquing a proposal or study may ask, "Are the findings relevant beyond the experimental condition?" Both the representitiveness of the subjects and the experimental settings must be considered when judging whether the findings can be applied elsewhere. Cook and Campbell (1979) identified six main factors that may jeopardize the external validity of a design: interaction effects of selection biases and the independent variable, the reactive effect of pretesting, the reactive effect of experimental procedures, multiple treatment interferences, interaction of history and treatment, and interaction of setting and treatment. When they are controlled, the researcher can achieve generalizability by replicating the study with different subjects, in different settings, and at different times. These six threats to external validity are described below.

- *Interaction of selection and treatment:* the effects obtained that are applicable only to the specific individuals who participated in the study. This threat to external validity is especially apt to occur the more unusual the requirements for participation. If participation is made as convenient and unextraordinary as possible, there is less likelihood of systematic recruitment factors operating that lead to results that apply only to the "very special people" who agree to participate.
- *Interaction of setting and treatment:* the effects obtained that are applicable only to the specific setting where the experiment is conducted. This threat also contains an element of selection bias because persons from some settings are more apt to agree to participate than those from others. The milieus of settings vary widely, with some being more innovative, more pleasant, and more competitive. The question is whether or not results obtained in one setting can be generalized to other settings that, because of their particular environments, would not or could not participate in the study.
- *Interaction of history and treatment:* the effects obtained that are applicable only to the specific time period within which the study is conducted. Unusual occurrences that coincide with a study period can make the extrapolation of results to other periods of time questionable. While the researcher can attempt to plan in a way that avoids obvious unusual occurrences, it is often impossible to avoid happenings that could make the findings unique to the study time period. Also, the generalization of findings to future time periods is always questionable. Replication of studies at different times is the logical approach to counteracting the interaction effect of history.

Cook and Campbell (1979) refer to additional threats to external validity that have been described by Campbell and Stanley (1963) as "threats to construct validity." Because most research texts continue to subsume "threats to construct validity" under "threats to external validity," these threats are listed and described below.

- *Reaction or interaction effect of pretesting:* following exposure to the pretest, the subjects no longer remain representative of the target population, which has not been pretested. Thus the findings cannot be generalized to the target population. This effect occurs because the nature of the pretest makes subjects aware of certain issues or events of which they would not otherwise be aware, causing them to respond to the treatment in a unique way.

• *Reactive effect of experimental procedures:* the effect produced by the procedures of the experiment that make the subjects who are exposed to these procedures no longer representative of the target population; this is commonly known as the "Hawthorne effect."

• *Multiple treatment interference:* effects produced by multiple exposures of subjects to a treatment, so that the results may be generalizable only to individuals who also receive the same multiple exposures to the treatment in the same sequence.

Causality. Experimental designs are used to test hypotheses of cause-and-effect relationships between variables; that is, when X occurs it is likely that Y will result. Although causal laws can never be proved, researchers proposing or critiquing experimental designs should be aware of the three criteria for causality (Selltiz, Wrightsman, & Cook, 1976, p. 115): (1) a temporal relationship, that is, the cause must precede the effect in time; (2) an empirical relationship, that is, there must be evidence that the independent variable and the dependent variable are associated; and (3) the relationship cannot be explained by the influence of a third variable (or spurious relationship). Some examples may serve to clarify these criteria: A correlational study in which the researcher proposes that X, decreased nurse responsiveness (as measured by amount of time taken to answer call lights) causes Y, increased number of patient complaints, fails to meet the criterion of a temporal relationship because it is *equally* possible that the effect (Y) may precede the cause (X). That is, increased complaining on the part of patients may lead nurses to stop responding efficiently, as they dread dealing with patient complaints and therefore delay unpleasant encounters by failing to respond to call lights.

A study suggesting that excessive trace elements such as aluminum (X) causes Alzheimer's disease (Y) would have to meet the criterion of an empirical relationship by demonstrating an association between the ingestion of aluminum and the presence of Alzheimer's disease using, for example, specimens from the hippocampus region of the brain on autopsy.

Finally, a nurse researcher who has observed a relationship between number of ice cream cones consumed (X) and number of drownings

(Y) cannot conclude there is a causal relationship between eating ice cream and drowning without taking into consideration a third spurious variable, Z (season of the year), that influences both X and Y. That is, there are more ice cream cones consumed in the warm summer months, and there are more drownings also, because more people go to the beach in the summer months as well. This somewhat humorous example illustrates an important point, that correlation is a necessary but insufficient condition for causality. However, knowledge gained about the relationship among variables using correlational designs can serve as the basis for the testing of causal relationships using experimental designs.

Only in true experimental designs can plausible alternative explanations for observed relationships be eliminated or discredited. This is because experimental designs have the highest internal validity and thus the greatest control over factors other than those advanced by the research hypotheses that might explain the findings. When a smaller number of plausible interpretations are available to account for the data, a theory is confirmed to a greater degree (Campbell & Stanley, 1963).

SUMMARY OF STRENGTHS AND WEAKNESSES

A major advantage of experimental designs is the degree of confidence they allow the researcher in inferring causal relationships. This is the case because true experiments have greater internal validity than other methodological approaches. A high degree of internal validity enables the researcher to rule out rival or alternative explanations to a causal interpretation. Establishing causal relationships is important to researchers because it enhances their ability to predict and therefore control phenomena. Despite these advantages, the proportion of experimental studies reported in the nursing literature remains relatively small, though experimental research conducted by nurses is increasing.

Experimental designs are not perfect. Among the limitations already noted are the number of potentially interesting research variables that are not within the researcher's purview to manipulate. Ethical concerns, organizational prohibitions, and human characteristics often interfere with the researcher's ability to control a number of variables experimentally. Moreover, the sample is usually not representative. In order to increase control of extraneous variables, the sample is often quite homogeneous prior to random assignment and therefore many replications may be required to achieve any generalizability.

Another design limitation, apparent in laboratory experiments especially, is their artificiality, and thus diminished external validity. Yet another compromise to generalizability is the "Hawthorne effect," or the reactive effects created by subjects' knowledge that they are participating in an experiment. Finally, many of the phenomena of interest to nursing are simply not yet well described and do not have an adequate theoretical base to be tested appropriately in an experimental mode. Rather, these phenomena are best approached in exploratory and/or descriptive studies that will generate hypotheses for experimental testing at a later stage in the development of nursing knowledge.

Research settings. Researchers frequently distinguish between "field experiments" and "laboratory experiments" based on the setting where the research is conducted. Field experiments are conducted in real-life settings, such as hospitals, that are particularly well suited to testing nursing phenomena. Realistic research settings contribute to the study's external validity, but field experiments often lack control of variance, as it is difficult to control extraneous environmental variables in real-life settings. Conversely, laboratory experiments are conducted in highly controlled, artificial settings in which the investigator has great control over all experimental conditions. Because of these characteristics, laboratory experiments usually contain less error variance and are more easily replicated than field studies. The artificiality of the research setting, while boosting the internal validity of the experiment, diminishes its generalizability and occasionally the impact of the experimental treatment as well. Both types of experiments are crucial to the generation of nursing knowledge. Both have inherent strengths and weaknesses that the researcher should consider when choosing a research setting. As with the choice of design, the choice of research setting (e.g., field or laboratory) should be determined by the nature of the research questions under consideration.

Sampling issues. In many experimental situations, subjects cannot be randomly selected from a defined population. In other words, a complete list of all persons in a population (the sampling frame) cannot be obtained from which a random sample can be drawn. Although probability sampling of subjects is ideal, and the best way to generalize research findings beyond the sample, the realities of clinical research, in particular, often prohibit random sampling. In experimental designs the use of random assignment provides control of sample variables by the random distribution of important characteristics to both experimental and control groups.

In many clinical experiments, subjects are selected on the basis of such variables as presence of a given disease or syndrome at a given point in time. All persons who meet selected inclusion criteria and who consent to participate are thus enrolled in the study. More often than not, subjects are selected sequentially as they arrive for a particular treatment. In these field settings it is frequently infeasible to locate and list the population in advance of subject selection. Moreover, in many cases the population is unknown.

Lack of probability sampling poses several methodological disadvantages. First, without random sampling it is difficult to generalize research findings beyond the sample. In addition, experimental designs employ rigorous control over many variables, making the sample unrepresentative of real-world cohorts and thus generalizations to the population questionable. Second, inferential statistics should be applied only to data obtained from probability samples. Parametric statistical procedures commonly used to analyze experimental results, such as analysis of variance, have a number of underlying assumptions that are best met through random sampling.

Third, only with probability sampling are researchers able to determine sample size according to how much sampling error (the differences between population values and sample values) they are willing to accept. In experimental designs without probability sampling, the desired sample size is dependent upon the number and type of variables under study. If subgroups within the sample are to be analyzed, the sample size often must be increased. Ns of 20-30 subjects per subdivision of the data (or each cell of a factorial design) are recommended, with the minimum being 10 per group. The researcher must ensure the generation of sufficient data for purposes of analysis through the testing of an adequate number of subjects. In general, and when economically feasible, large samples are preferable to small samples. Data from larger samples usually are more reliable, more representative of the population of interest, have fewer sampling errors, and provide more statistical power for purposes of analysis. Increased sample size also decreases the probability of type I (alpha) and type II (beta) errors in hypothesis testing. (See the discussion of hypothesis testing, below.)

Finally, larger samples permit the principle of randomization to function better in the distribution of sample characteristics between groups.

Measurement of outcomes in experimental design. Selection of poor outcome measures (dependent variables) can undermine a nursing research project. Outcome measurement includes four issues: (1) relevant outcome variables, (2) validity, (3) reliability, and (4) systematic biases.

Relevant outcome variables are crucial for answering causal research questions. In the example of depressed patients randomly assigned to an experimental nursing intervention designed to treat depression, one obvious criterion measure of effectiveness of the intervention is whether treated patients improve on measures of depression. There are a number of ways to measure depression, ranging from indirect physiological parameters such as MHPG levels in urine to self-report instruments such as the Beck Depression Inventory. Which outcome variables are most relevant depends upon the study's theoretical framework, the objectives of the intervention, and the research questions addressed. In this example, the nurse researcher might also be interested in recidivisim and/or suicide rates, vocational adjustment following the intervention, and family attitudes toward the patient. To measure these diverse aftercare variables the nurse researcher might use structured observations or interviews and archival data. The point is that whether and how these variables are measured depends upon the objectives of the particular intervention. The independent variable and its outcome criteria must be correlated in the theoretical framework. For example, if the nursing intervention to alleviate depression is cognitive restructuring, then a dependent variable that captures cognitive changes is most appropriate. Similarly, if an intervention is psychopharmacological in nature for purposes of altering selected catacholamines, then a physiological measure of those catacholamines or their breakdown products is most relevant.

Often a variety of data collection methods is required in order to assess all the relevant outcome measures. If the intervention is truly effective, and the theoretical framework sound, then differences should be found on all reliable and valid outcome measures. Further, because these measures often involve different methods of assessment (see the discussion of triangulation, below), the nurse researcher can have increased confidence in the findings. This is because the more numerous and independent the ways in which the experimental effect is shown, the less plausible alternative explanations or rival hypotheses become (Campbell & Stanley, 1963).

The employment of measures that have demonstrated reliability and validity is critical to the success of any experiment. For an in-depth discussion of these issues, see Chapter 12 of this volume, "Methodological Studies: Instrument Development," by Merle Mishel.

Validity refers to whether a particular instrument actually measures the construct it is designed to assess (Carmines & Zeller, 1979). In the example of an experimental nursing intervention to treat depression, if an *invalid* measure of depression is used to assess patient outcome, then the researcher might falsely conclude that the intervention is effective or ineffective. Because of the instrument's lack of validity, scores would not be indicative of any true changes in depression that occurred due to the intervention. An invalid measure could be measuring some other property, such as powerlessness.

In selecting measures to use in any experiment, the researcher should carefully review the validity evidence for the measure. Mishel's chapter provides an excellent description of the different forms of validity employed in evaluating measurement instruments, including self-evident measures such as face and content validity, pragmatic measures or criterion-related validity (both concurrent and predictive), and construct validity. Construct validity deals with validation of the theory or construct underlying an experimental study. Ideally, experimental designs should use instruments with established construct validity. However, the multitrait, multimethod techniques used to establish construct validity are complex, and more often than not experiments are conducted using tools that have not yet achieved this highest level of validation.

Certain instruments may be valid only for selected populations or age groups. For example, if our nursing intervention was for treatment of the depressed *elderly*, then standard measures of depression widely used with younger age groups might not be valid for this study (Kane & Kane, 1981). Failure to use age-validated criteria could result in changes in cognitive abilities and physiological processes being labeled as pathological when in fact they are normal consequences of aging. Thus it is critical that measures of depression be validated for the elderly before they are used in this study.

Reliability is concerned with the accuracy (consistency, stability, and repeatability) of a measure in representing the true score of the subject being assessed on a particular dimension. Mishel's chapter presents an in-depth discussion of the ways to conceptualize and evaluate a measure's reliability, including tests of stability such as test-retest, tests for equivalence such as alternate forms, and tests of internal consistency, which assure that the concept is measured consistently throughout the instrument.

It is important to employ reliable measures in any experimental study, as unreliable measures may not be sensitive or accurate enough to detect differences in the experimental versus the control group. That is, the effect of measurement error (discussed earlier in this chapter in the section on *control of variance*) is to attenuate or reduce the differences between groups, which can undermine efforts to demonstrate the effectiveness of a particular intervention. In general, reliability coefficients should be at least 0.70. The reliability coefficient is determined by what proportion of the test variance is *nonerror* variance.

Biases in measurement can be minimized by using more than one method of measurement. The use of multiple methods of data collection and sources (*triangulation* of the measurement process) is recommended to ensure assessing the range of relevant outcome measures for a particular experiment. This approach, using multiple methods of assessment, also helps to counteract systematic biases that may be present in some measures. Often, patients or staff may be biased in their assessments, out of a desire to see a particular intervention succeed. These biases can lead to false conclusions of effectiveness on the part of the researcher. Employing a variety of data collection methods will help to counteract this type of bias.

It is important to use data collectors who are "blind" to (that is, unknowledgeable about) which subjects received the experimental condition and which are controls. This means that the same research assistant who delivers the nursing intervention should not collect the outcome data related to that intervention. Additional personnel who do *not* hold preconceptions should be employed to collect the outcome data. An experimental ideal in terms of decreasing bias is the *double-blind* procedure, in which neither the subject nor the observer knows the group to which the subject is assigned. Yet another approach to decreasing bias is to assign more than one data collector for each subject and then calculate interrater agreements. It is often sufficient to check interrater reliability on only a random 10% of all data sets.

In experimental designs the data collection methods are highly structured, the approach to data collection is deductive and theory testing, and the researcher controls the variables and the experimental conditions. A wide variety of data collection methods are acceptable, and multiple methods of assessment are encouraged, as long as the conditions and measurements are identical for all subjects. This high degree of structure is usually an asset when it comes to data preparation and analysis.

Hypothesis testing. Experimental research is theory-testing research, and, whereas experimental findings can never be used to "prove" a theory, successful theories avoid disconfirmation. Hypotheses are statements concerning predicted relationships among the variables under study that link a study's theoretical framework to experimental realities. Hypotheses provide overall direction to any experiment and guide every aspect of the research process, including sampling, data collection, and analysis. The components of a hypothesis are examined in detail in Brink and Wood (1983, pp. 67-73). In general, a well-written hypothesis (1) is neutral in tone rather than value-laden, (2) precisely and parsimoniously identifies the independent and dependent variables, and (3) identifies how the dependent variable is measured. The research hypothesis in experimental designs should be derived from a theory, must specify the predicted relationship between two or more variables, and must be testable; that is, the variables specified must be measurable. The *null hypothesis* is set up for purposes of possible rejection. It is an arbitrary convention and the hypothesis that is tested statistically. The null hypothesis postulates that any differences found between the experimental and control groups would be due to chance alone or to sampling errors. The *research* (or working) *hypothesis* states the researcher's expectations, identifying the factors in a causal relationship that are believed to account for the findings. Rejecting the null hypothesis suggests support for the research hypothesis. Researchers can commit two types of errors in accepting or rejecting the null hypothesis. *Type I error* (alpha) occurs when the null hypothesis is rejected and it is true; that is, no differences actually exist in the data. Alpha errors are best avoided by choosing a conservative (alpha = .05) level of significance. *Type II error* (beta) occurs when the null hypothesis is accepted falsely; that is, the researcher concludes that no difference exists when it actually does.

Data analysis. Tests of hypotheses are one form of analysis experimenters engage in. Which statistical test is selected depends upon what the hypothesis predicts, the level of measurement, and assumptions related to the data. In the classic experimental design, a comparison of two sample means (the posttest data for the control and experimental groups) is made to determine whether or not the independent variable "made a difference." The null hypothesis under test is that the two means are the same (H_0: $\bar{X}_1 = \bar{X}_2$), and the alternative or research hypothesis is that the two means differ (H_1: $\bar{X}_1 > \bar{X}_2$, $\bar{X}_1 < \bar{X}_2$, or $\bar{X}_1 \neq \bar{X}_2$). Statistical procedures such as a *t*-test for differences between two groups or analysis of variance (ANOVA) for differences among multiple groups can be used to test these hypotheses. A significant F statistic using the ANOVA procedure indicates that the "among-group" variance is larger than the "within-group" variance. Because these tests are based on comparisons of sample means, the level of measurement must be at least interval level. These parametric tests assume (1) that the data are normally distributed and (2) that the variances of the data are similar. Both the *t*-test and ANOVA have nonparametric or "distribution-free" counterparts including the Mann-Whitney U test and the Kruskall-Wallis one-way ANOVA for ordinal data, respectively. Siegel (1956) provides an excellent reference on nonparametric procedures.

It can be misleading to compare *t*-tests on a before-and-after basis without first comparing initial differences between the control and experimental groups. If the researcher has collected pretreatment data on both the experimental and control group using the same outcome measure, then these pretest measures can be employed as covariates in an analysis of covariance (ANCOVA) procedure. The effect of this procedure is blocking or "leveling out" of the pretest scores and the adjustment of posttest scores to compensate for initial lack of equivalence between groups. Thus ANCOVA adjusts for initial differences between groups and for the correlation between means. A more complete discussion of ANCOVA appears in Chapter 3 of this volume, on quasi-experimental designs.

PILOT STUDY

A pilot study is strongly recommended before the conduct of any major experiment. This preliminary investigation or "trial run," using a limited number of subjects, permits the researcher to test and possibly reshape or add hypotheses. The proposed data collection and analysis procedure can also be evaluated and changed as needed. Unanticipated problems arise during the course of almost any study, and a pilot study enables the researcher to identify and deal with these before the major study is sabotaged. The value of pilot studies is emphasized by the fact that grants submitted to the National Institute of Health are rarely awarded without evidence of pilot data.

ETHICAL CONSIDERATIONS

The protection of the rights of all human and animal subjects is the obligation of every researcher, and these rights are protected by federal law. Perhaps the most important concern for human subjects comes in the area of informed consent. All subjects who participate in an experimental study must clearly understand its purpose, procedures, the researcher's expectations of them as subjects, the length of the experiment, and projected use of the data. Researchers must also inform subjects of expected benefits as well as risks they may incur as a result of participation in the study. These risks are interpreted to be psychosocial as well as physical in nature. Researchers must further provide adequate treatment and referral mechanisms for participants should injury develop during the course of the experiment. Participation must be voluntary and subjects must be assured of their right to withdraw from the study at any time without prejudice. True informed consent means the researcher cannot withhold information or deceive subjects in any way, even if knowledge of the research purpose or methods might affect their response. Nor can subjects be coerced in any way to participate—for example, by intimating that needed treatment might be withheld.

Of particular concern in experimental designs, which typically employ a control or comparison group, is the notion that the research approach should not deprive control subjects of necessary care or information. Experimental studies that employ a placebo drug or effect must therefore be carefully scrutinized. As in other methodologies, the researcher using an experimental design must avoid an invasion of subjects' privacy, assure subjects of anonymity or confidentiality, and inform them of plans for publishing findings of the study without identification of individual participants (American Nurses Association, 1968; Armiger, 1977; Jacobsen, 1973).

CRITIQUING EXPERIMENTS

Although experimental designs provide for the most rigorous tests of hypotheses, no one design is perfect, and many experiments reported in the literature are flawed and subject to question. Perhaps the experiment was not well conceptualized to begin with, or perhaps the experimental conditions were not carefully controlled, the analyses imprecise, or interpretations rendered that went beyond the scope of the data. Especially in field settings, adequate control over all variables is extremely difficult to achieve.

Batey (1971) has classified experimental pitfalls into three major areas: conceptual, empirical, and interpretive. Conceptual problems most frequently encountered have to do with poorly defined or inconsequential research problems, and a lack of congruence between study variables and the theoretical "roots" of the study. Hypotheses may be poorly stated, or it may be inappropriate to be testing the hypotheses altogether. That is, perhaps exploratory (Level I) or descriptive (Level II) questions (Brink & Wood, 1983) are better suited to the phenomena under study, and it is premature to test hypotheses and attempt to establish cause-and-effect relationships among the variables.

Empirical problems center largely on control of variance issues, discussed earlier in this chapter. Without adequate control over extraneous variables, the researcher cannot be confident that it was the independent variable(s) that was (were) responsible for any observed changes in the dependent variable(s), an issue of the internal validity of the study. The external validity, or generalizability of findings, is also subject to criticism. For example, if characteristics of either the sample or population are unknown, inferences from one to the other may not be valid.

Problems of interpretation of the data may arise from a variety of sources, including inappropriate analysis procedures and lack of congruence with the study's theoretical framework. It is not uncommon for beginning researchers, in particular, to make assertions that have no basis in the research findings (that is, that go beyond the data) or to fail to consider adequately the study's limitations (e.g., small sample size or measurement errors) when developing inferences from results. In experimental designs, which are theory testing in nature, the supporting theoretical framework should guide all interpretations of the data. It is essential to report data that support, as well as disconfirm, the null hypotheses. Reviewers may also question whether human subjects' rights were adequately protected in the experiment and whether the merit of the study was proportionate to the risks incurred.

Although a number of approaches to critiquing experimental studies are available, Binder (1981, pp. 158-159) has developed a comprehensive criterion checklist for critiquing nursing research using experimental designs. The checklist is based on Batey's three-part classification scheme. Many of the pitfalls and issues related to the conduct and analysis of experimental studies discussed thus far will become clearer in this final section, where three designs are examined in relation to actual nursing studies.

USE OF EXPERIMENTAL DESIGNS IN NURSING RESEARCH

In reviewing the classic experimental design (pretest, posttest, control group), subjects are randomly assigned to the experimental and control groups.

$$\text{RA} \quad \frac{O_1 \; X \; O_2 \; (Ex)}{O_3 \quad\;\; O_4 \; (Con)}$$

where RA = random assignment, O = observations, Ex = experimental group, and Con = control group.

Subjects are pretested on the dependent variable (O_1, O_3) before subjects in the experimental group receive the experimental manipulation (X). Both groups are subsequently posttested (O_2, O_4) and the differences between their scores on the dependent variable are analyzed using a *t*-test or F test. This design has many advantages. First, it is simple, and random assignment of subjects helps to assure that the groups are equivalent at the beginning of the study. The comparison group controls for threats to internal validity such as history (the influence of events that might occur during the study, and could affect the dependent variable) and maturation (processes occurring within the subjects themselves as a function of the passage of time). As both groups are pretested, any sensitizing effects of the pretest should be equally distributed (controlling for the effects of testing). However, results can be generalized only to similarly pretested groups, which decreases the study's external validity.

A number of variations on the classic experimental design exist. This design can be extended to more than one independent variable, as in the Eland (1982) example below, and to more than one measurement of the dependent variable(s), as noted in the Layton (1979) example that follows.

Factorial Designs

Classical experimental design allows the manipulation of a single independent variable at a time, holding all other conditions constant. Frequently, phenomena of interest to nurses are more complex than the classical design permits, and factors may *interact* to produce behaviors of interest to nurse researchers. As noted earlier, *factorial designs* permit more than one independent variable to be manipulated at a time, and thus allow the testing of multiple hypotheses simultaneously. Further, interaction effects between variables are revealed, making factorial designs an important variation on the classical experimental design. Although the example used in this chapter is a 2 × 2 factorial design, factorial experiments can be conducted with three or more independent variables (known as factors). Each factor must have two or more levels. Thus when new factors are added more hypotheses can be tested simultaneously. Concurrently, the interpretation of main effects and interaction effects becomes more complex with the addition of new factors. Factorial designs are also referred to as "levels by treatment" designs. When one of the factors cannot be manipulated, such as sex of subjects, it is referred to as a *blocking variable*. The design that incorporates the blocking variable is known as a *randomized block design*.

Design 1: 2 × 2 Factorial

The purpose of this study was to investigate the effects of two separate nursing interventions on the amount of pain experienced by prekindergarten children undergoing a routine DPT immunization (Eland, 1982). A 2 × 2 factorial design was used to test the two nursing interventions. Intervention 1 altered the transmission of pain messages from the skin surface by spraying a skin coolant, Frigiderm, on the injection site immediately prior to the injection. One half of the subjects had Frigiderm sprayed on the injection site prior to the injection, while the other half had aerosol air sprayed on their legs prior to injection. Intervention 2 altered the processing and interpretation of injection pain by giving cognitive information. One-half of the subjects were told by the nurse prior to injection, "I'm going to spray something on your leg before your shot that will not hurt, that will make your leg feel cool, and the spray will make this shot hurt less than other shots you've had." The other half of the subjects were told only that the nurse was "going to spray something on their leg before their shot." The sample consisted of 20 male and 20 female prekindergarteners. There were 5 males and 5 females included in each of the two levels of the two treatment groups. Children scheduled for physical exams during a one-month period were stratified by the variables of sex and nurse who would give the injection. Each child was then *randomly assigned* to one of the treatment groups. The dependent variable, amount of pain experienced with the injection, was assessed using the Eland color tool, with its 4-point pain scale (0 = no pain to 3 = severe pain). Subjects in Group A received Frigiderm and cognitive information, those in Group B received air and cognitive information, those in Group C received Frigiderm but no cognitive information, and those in Group D received air and no cognitive information (see Figure 2.1).

A two-factor analysis of variance was used to answer the research question. The ANOVA test dimensions consisted of (1) a *main effect* for type of spray, (2) a *main effect* for type of cognitive information, and (3) the *interaction effects* of spray and cognitive information. The main effect for type of spray was significant ($p = .029$). The main effect for cognitive information and the interaction effects of spray and cognitive information did not reach significance ($p = .521$ and $p = .337$, respectively), suggesting that Frigiderm used before the injection resulted in significant pain reduction regardless of the type of information given to the child about the spray.

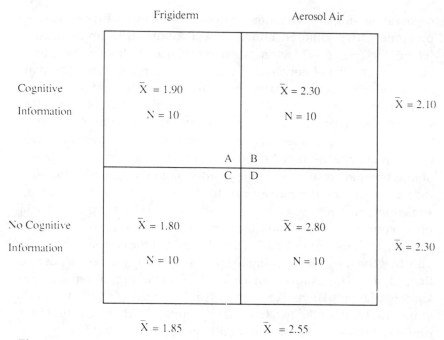

Figure 2.1. Amount of Pain Experienced by Prekindergarten Children During Routine DPT Immunizations

Design 2:
Multiple Treatment Groups—Repeated Measures Design

This experiment tested various combinations of modeling, labeling, and videotaped rehearsal to teach empathy to upper-division baccalaureate nursing students (Layton, 1979). There were four experimental groups: (1) modeling alone (X_1) , (2) modeling and labeling (X_2), (3) modeling and rehearsal (X_3), and (4) modeling and labeling and rehearsal (X_4). A fifth group served as a no-treatment control (C). This design incorporates multiple experimental groups that receive different treatments. Control is present in the sense of a formal comparison and the notion that a control group is always the "no-treatment" group is not absolute.

	Time 1	Time 2
X_1	0_1	0_2
X_2	0_3	0_4
X_3	0_5	0_6
X_4	0_7	0_8
C	0_9	0_{10}

Each subject was posttested on two occasions, immediately after treatment and three weeks later. A repeated measures design with time as a variable was employed, using student volunteers from the six junior and senior courses (N = 56). Assignment was randomized within the courses rather than within the total group of subjects to equalize systematic differences because of class level and prior learning experiences. Empathy, the dependent variable, was measured in three ways: (1) empathy test completed by subjects, (2) evaluation of a student-client interview using (a) the Barrett-Lennard Relationships Inventory and (b) the Carkhuff Empathetic Understanding in Interpersonal Processes Scale. On the second posttest an alternate form of the empathy test was used, otherwise all measurements were the same. Data were analyzed using multivariate analyses of variance. First, a repeated measures analysis of treatment by time was conducted, followed by separate analysis of the two posttest sessions. Findings for the total group of subjects were not significant, but when results of junior nursing students were analyzed separately, they were significant for treatment and interaction effects, especially on the Carkhuff scale.

Thus the modeling intervention appeared to produce a change in junior, but not senior, students. Regarding treatment effects, Scheffé post hoc procedures indicated that only the groups receiving modeling and rehearsal (X_3) performed better than the no-treatment control group. Modeling alone (X_1) and modeling and labeling (X_2) were not effective treatments—rehearsal was the only effective condition in this study.

Design 3: Solomon Four-Group Design

One of the most rigorous designs in terms of control of threats to both internal and external validity is the Solomon four-group design (Campbell & Stanley, 1963, p. 24). Subjects are randomly assigned to one of the four groups to promote statistical equivalence at the outset of the experiment. Lines 1 and 2 (pretested experimental and pretested control groups) control for the effects of history and maturation. Line 3 (unpretested experimental group) controls for the effects of pretesting, and the fourth line (unpretested control) controls for contemporaneous effects occurring between pre- and posttesting periods. Though a rigorous design, the Solomon four-group design is seldom employed in nursing research for a number of reasons. First, the four groups re-

quire a large number of homogeneous subjects. Second, conducting
the four groups concurrently to avoid temporal extraneous variables
is demanding, and usually requires multiple investigators and a great
deal of coordination of research activities. Third, the four groups do
not produce four complete sets of data, leading to a more complex
statistical analysis, as illustrated in the research example below:

$$
\begin{array}{cccc}
 & O_1 & X & O_2 \\
RA & O_3 & & O_4 \\
 & & X & O_5 \\
 & & & O_6
\end{array}
$$

Silva (1979) used the Solomon four-group design to test the effects
of orientation information on spouses' anxieties and attitudes toward
hospitalization and surgery. The theoretical base for her study was
cognitive dissonance theory. A total of 48 subjects (spouses of patients,
$N = 12$ per group) were randomly assigned to one of four groups: (a)
orientation information, pretest and posttest (line 1), (b) no orientation information, pretest and posttest (line 2), (c) orientation information, posttest only (line 3), and (d) no orientation information, posttest only (line 4). The two dependent variables of anxiety and attitudes
toward hospitalization and surgery were measured using Spielberger
et al.'s State Anxiety Inventory and the Spouses' Perception Scale,
developed by the researcher. Data analysis involved three tests. A 2
$\times$ 2 factorial analysis of variance tested the presence or absence of
pretesting and orientation information. Pretest scores were additionally
used as the covariate in a one-dimensional analysis of covariance with
homogeneity of regression test. Finally, chi-square tests were performed on 2 $\times$ 3 frequency contingency tables (pretest groups $\times$ anxiety
$\times$ attitude).

Data supported the hypothesis that spouses given orientation information would experience less anxiety than those not receiving information for the Spouse Questionnaire, but *not* for the State Anxiety Inventory. Spouses who received orientation information did exhibit
better attitudes toward hospitalization and surgery than spouses in the
control group. It is interesting to note that both the main and inter-
active effects of pretesting were insignificant.

CONCLUSION

The purposes of research designs are to answer research questions in a valid manner and to control sources of variance. Experimental designs are the most precise method researchers can employ to generate evidence in support of postulated causal relationships among variables. Experimental research should be well grounded theoretically and based upon cumulative research findings. In experimental studies, three elements are essential: randomization, control, and manipulation of the independent variable(s) by the investigator. Within these criteria, there are a number of variations on the classic experimental design that permit use of multiple groups, multiple independent variables, and multiple measurements of the dependent variable over time. Although experimental designs offer the most rigorous control over extraneous variables and therefore have strong internal validity, they are by no means always the ideal choice for answering a research question. Pragmatic considerations such as cost, time, generalizability, and factors associated with the research setting must also be evaluated when one is choosing a research strategy. In general, however, experimental designs are considered to be the most powerful approach available to nurse researchers in that they maximize the effect of the independent variable, minimize error, and control extraneous variables better than any other research mode.

REFERENCES

American Nurses Association. (1986). The nurse in research: ANA guidelines on ethical values. *Nursing Research, 17*, 104-107.

Armiger, Sister B. (1977). Ethics of nursing research: Profile, principles, perspectives. *Nursing Research, 26*, 330-336.

Batey, M. W. (1971). Conceptualizing the research process. *Nursing Research, 20*, 296.

Binder, D. M. (1981). Critique: Experimental study. In S. D. Krampitz & N. Pavlovich (Eds.), *Readings for nursing research*. Chicago: Rand McNally.

Brink, P. J., & Wood, M. J. (1983). *Basic steps in planning nursing research: From question to proposal* (2nd ed.). Monterey, CA: Wadsworth Health Sciences.

Campbell, D. T., & Stanley, J. (1963). *Experimental and quasi-experimental designs for research*. Chicago: Rand McNally.

Carmines, E. G., & Zeller, R. A. (1979). *Reliability and validity assessment*. Beverly Hills, CA: Sage.

Cook, T. D., & Campbell, D. T. (Eds.). (1979). *Quasi-experimentation: Design and analysis issues for field settings*. Chicago: University of Chicago Press.

Eland, J. M. (1982). Minimizing injection pain associated with prekindergarten immunization. *Issues in Comprehensive Pediatric Nursing, 5*(5/6), 361-372.

Isaac, S., & Michael, W. B. (1971). *Handbook of research and evaluation.* San Diego, CA: EDITS.

Jacobsen, S. F. (1973). Ethical issues on experimentation with human subjects. *Nursing Forum, 12,* 58-71.

Kane, R. A., & Kane, R. L. (1981). *Assessing the elderly: A practical guide to measurement.* Lexington, MA: Lexington.

Kerlinger, F. N. (1973). *Foundations of behavioral research* (2nd ed.). New York: Holt, Rinehart & Winston.

Kuzma, J. W. (1984). *Basic statistics for the health sciences.* Palo Alto, CA: Mayfield.

Layton, J. M. (1979). The use of modeling to teach empathy to nursing students. *Research in Nursing and Health, 2,* 163-176.

Selltiz, C., Wrightsman, L. S., & Cook, S. W. (1976). *Research model in social relations* (3rd ed.). New York: Holt, Rinehart & Winston.

Sherwood, C. D., Morris, J. N., & Sherwood, S. (1975). A multivariate, nonrandomized matching technique for studying the impact of social interventions. In E. L. Struening & M. Guttentag (Eds.), *Handbook of evaluation research* (Vol. 1, pp. 183-224). Beverly Hills, CA: Sage.

Siegel, S. (1956). *Nonparametric statistics for the behavioral sciences.* New York: McGraw-Hill.

Silva, M. C. (1979). Effects of orientation information on spouses' anxieties and attitudes toward hospitalization and surgery. *Research in Nursing and Health, 2,* 127-136.

Spector, P. E. (1981). *Research designs.* Beverly Hills, CA: Sage.

3. Quasi-Experimental Designs

Meridean L. Maas
Kathleen C. Buckwalter

Very often in the "real world" of nursing research the use of the true experiment is not a viable option. Much of the research that is relevant for nursing practice and for the development of nursing science must be conducted in natural settings. The researcher is often not allowed control of the treatment variable and cannot achieve randomization because of ethical considerations, institutional policies, or other situational factors. When these circumstances are present, the nurse researcher can look to quasi-experiments for alternative research strategies rather than forgo the systematic study of many phenomena for which the use of an experimental design is not possible. Quasi-experiments are sufficiently probing to be worth employing, especially when more efficient probes are not possible (Campbell & Stanley, 1963). They are appropriate for Level III questions (Brink & Wood, 1983), which aim to explain why a relationship exists, and are very often the strategy that the nurse in the clinical field setting will use to test theories of causal relationships.

In some circumstances randomization may be the source of problems that the researcher would not want to introduce into the study. For example, the nursing administration of a hospital may want to study the effects of flex time on staff nurses' job performance. Staff nurse subjects are drawn from two different patient care units and randomly assigned to experimental and control groups. A problem that can arise when this method is used is referred to by Cook and Campbell (1979) as "resentful demoralization." Because the experimental and control subjects work daily in close proximity, nurses in the control group who are not allowed flex time may become resentful of the nurses in the experimental group and experience demoralization. In this situation the objectives of the investigation would be better served by selecting nurses from one unit for the experimental group and nurses from another unit for the control group. This is so even though there may be a number of differences between the two groups of nurses and the patient care units that will introduce sources of variance in job performance.

Quasi-experimental designs also represent important strategies for nurse researchers who plan an experimental study and experience nonrandom dropout of subjects assigned to experimental and control groups. When this occurs, the two groups can no longer be assumed to be equivalent on all factors other than the treatment. Thus the initial experimental design has become a quasi-experimental design. When conducting experimental studies the nurse researcher must carefully evaluate subject attrition and will be equipped to continue the test of causal hypotheses if knowledgeable about the quasi-experimental strategies that can be employed secondarily.

QUASI-EXPERIMENTAL DESIGNS

Quasi-experiments, as the name implies, are designs that resemble true experiments. Quasi-experimental designs partially employ the control over threats to internal validity that are provided by true experimental designs. The inability to achieve experimental controls in field experiments led to the development of quasi-experimental designs and to special controls if random assignment was not possible (Cook & Campbell, 1979). Quasi-experiments are experiments that do not have equivalent groups created by random assignment or that do not have control groups for comparison so that the researcher can infer change due to a treatment effect. Rather, comparisons must be made with nonequivalent groups or with periodic measurement on the same group that may be different due to a number of variables extraneous to the causal variable of interest. Thus the major problem facing the researcher who uses quasi-experimental designs is in distinguishing the effects that are due to the treatment from those that are due to uncontrolled extraneous variables.

Quasi-experimental designs can be described in two general categories (Cook & Campbell, 1979). *Nonequivalent group designs* are those in which dependent variable measures are obtained for an experimental and a comparison group (nonrandomly assigned) before and after introduction of the independent variable to the experimental group. *Interrupted time-series designs* are those in which the independent variable effects are inferred by comparing measures of the dependent variable obtained at multiple time intervals with multiple dependent variable measures obtained after introduction of the independent variable. The basic time-series design uses a single group of subjects. There are several variations of each of these two basic quasi-experimental designs. Campbell and Stanley (1963) and Cook and Campbell (1979) are the seminal works that detail the numerous variations of these basic designs that are available to the field researcher. Knowledge of these basic designs and the assumptions underlying them is critical to the effective use of the variations of quasi-experimental designs. Discussion of these variations will be limited to those most likely to be employed by nurse researchers.

ADVANTAGES AND DISADVANTAGES OF QUASI-EXPERIMENTAL DESIGNS

Strengths

The major advantage of quasi-experimental designs is their usefulness as strategies for testing causal hypotheses in field settings. Many research questions of interest to nurse investigators are not amenable to random assignment of subjects to experimental and control conditions. Quasi-experimental designs are not only practical and feasible, they are directly relevant to the "real nursing world." Quasi-experiments represent essential alternative strategies to extend the scope of nursing research and to prevent the loss of causal tests due to the deterioration of true experiments in field settings. Quasi-experiments provide a systematic framework for answering questions that might otherwise be left to subjective analysis, trial and error, or conclusions drawn from compromised experiments in which rival causal hypotheses have not been explicitly evaluated. Further, quasi-experiments enhance generalizability over true experiments. Although replication

is needed for maximum generalizability, quasi-experiments are ordinarily less intrusive upon conditions in natural settings, less artificial,
and more apt to be representative of the real world of nursing practice.

Weaknesses

Quasi-experimental designs, by definition, lack the controls inherent
in experimental designs, such as variance in the dependent variable
from sources other than the treatment variable. The principal purposes
of designs for testing causal relationships are to provide controls to
maximize the effect of the independent variable on the dependent
variable, to minimize the effects of extraneous variables on the dependent variable, and to minimize measurement error. The major short-
coming of the quasi-experimental design is its lack of control over
extraneous sources of variance that threaten the conclusion that the
treatment variable produced the measured changes in the criterion
variable (Campbell & Stanley, 1963). Because of the lack of random
assignment, the experimental and comparison subjects may be different
in some systematic way. These differences may then be the reason for
any measured differences in the criterion variable that are obtained.
It is essential, therefore, to analyze actively and attempt to rule out
other causal explanations for the findings before concluding that the
treatment variable produced the measured differences in the criterion
variable.

The rival variables that may cause the group differences on the
criterion variable are described as "threats to internal validity" and
"threats to external validity" (generalizability of results) (Campbell &
Stanley, 1963; Cook & Campbell, 1979). See Chapter 2 for a description of these variables and the research example that follows for an
application of these principles.

CRITERIA FOR EVALUATING DESIGNS

Threats to Internal Validity

Campbell and Stanley (1963) present eight types of extraneous variables that potentially jeopardize internal validity. Cook and Campbell
(1979) describe twelve threats to internal validity that need to be considered for different types of designs. The sources of extraneous

variance that can confound the effects of the treatment on the criterion, if not controlled, that are especially critical for the evaluation of the adequacy of quasi-experimental designs are (1) history, (2) maturation, (3) testing, (4) instrumentation, (5) statistical regression, (6) selection, (7) experimental mortality, (8) selection maturation interaction, (9) selection-history interaction, (10) diffusion or imitation of treatments, (11) compensatory equalization of treatments, and (12) compensatory rivalry by respondents receiving less desirable treatments. See Chapter 2 for a description of these variables.

Threats to External Validity

Cook and Campbell (1979) assert that the external validity of a design is reflected in the design's ability to produce outcomes that can be generalized to particular target persons, settings, and times, and that can be generalized across types of persons, settings, and times. Thus they emphasize the need to distinguish clearly between generalizing to a specific target population and generalizing across populations in evaluating the external validity of an experimental design.

In other words, research results obtained with a randomly selected representative sample could be generalized to the target population, but not necessarily to specific subgroups of the population. Although both aspects of generalizability are relevant to assessing external validity, Cook and Campbell (1979) focus more on generalizing across subpopulations. This is because random sampling for representativeness that would allow generalization to a target population is not often done in field research. In addition, experiments that employ representative sampling with random assignment invariably experience attrition, so that when the research is completed the sample no longer represents the same population. For these reasons external validity is considered to be strengthened more by multiple small studies with nonrandom samples even if a single study could be implemented with a representative sample.

Thus the analyses of the ability to generalize across various subpopulations are basically tests of statistical interactions (Cook & Campbell, 1979). The different magnitudes of effects across types of subjects, settings, and other subpopulations must be specified in order to explain these different effects. The threats to external validity are expressed as the following statistical interaction effects: (1) interaction of selection and treatment, (2) interaction of setting and treatment, (3) interaction of history and treatment, (4) reaction or interaction effect of pretesting, (5) reactive effects of experimental procedures, and (6) multiple treatment interference. See Chapter 2, on experimental design, for a description of these effects.

A NURSING RESEARCH EXAMPLE

Maas and Buckwalter (1985) designed a study to evaluate experimentally the effects of a special Alzheimer's unit at the Iowa Veterans Home (IVH) in Marshalltown, Iowa. The study is systematically assessing the effects of the therapeutically structured unit environment on Alzheimer's (AD) patient functioning, selected staff responses, and family attitudes toward care, as well as the cost-effectiveness of the unit. AD patients are assigned either to a unit with physical environment, programs, staffing, and staff training designed for care of the AD patient or to a traditional integrated patient care unit. Patients are being followed for twelve months to gather baseline data and for eighteen months after exposure to the experimental conditions. The specific aim of the study is to answer the following questions:

(1) Are there slower rates of deterioration in terms of functional and cognitive abilities for AD patients on the special care unit?
(2) Are there fewer falls for the AD patients on the special care unit?
(3) Are fewer medications used for AD patients on the special care unit?
(4) Is it more cost-effective to care for AD patients on a specialized care unit as opposed to the traditional approach of caring for them on integrated long-term care units?
(5) Do staff report more satisfaction with their jobs, less burnout, and less stress when they care for AD patients on a special care unit?
(6) Are family members' perceptions of AD patients' care more positive if patients are cared for on the special care unit?

Measures of each of the effect variables were collected every other month throughout the study period. The design for this research is illustrated in Figure 3.1. There is no symbol R that indicates random assignment to the comparison groups. Rather, the dashed line separating the parallel rows indicates comparison groups that are not equated by random assignment. The X notation indicates introduction of the treatment variable and O indicates measurements of the dependent variable(s) (Campbell & Stanley, 1963). Both of the basic nonequivalent groups and time-series designs are embedded in Figure 3.1.

$$O_1 \quad O_2 \quad O_3 \quad O_4 \quad X \quad O_5 \quad O_6 \quad O_7 \quad O_8$$

$$O_1 \quad O_2 \quad O_3 \quad O_4 \qquad\quad O_5 \quad O_6 \quad O_7 \quad O_8$$

Figure 3.1. Design to Evaluate the Effects of a Special Alzheimer's Unit
SOURCE: Cook and Campbell (1979). Reprinted by permission.
NOTE: X = introduction of the treatment (independent variable); O = observations or measures; dashed line = nonrandom assignment to groups/nonequivalent groups; numerical subscripts = same measures at different times.

NONEQUIVALENT GROUPS DESIGNS

In the basic nonequivalent groups design, one group of individuals is designated to receive a program, service or treatment (experimental group) and a second group of individuals is designated as a control group. This design is called the *untreated control group design with pretest and posttest* (Cook & Campbell, 1979). Figure 3.2. presents the schematic of the basic nonequivalent groups design, using the codes defined in Chapter 2.

$$O_1 \qquad X \qquad O_2$$

$$O_1 \qquad\qquad O_2$$

Figure 3.2. The Nonequivalent Groups Design
SOURCE: Cook and Campbell (1979). Reprinted by permission.
NOTE: See note to Figure 3.1. for explanation of figure elements.

This design is often used in field research where variable relationships characterizing human subjects are tested. The design is identical to the classical experimental pretest-posttest control group design except that subjects are *not* randomly assigned to the experimental and control groups. Because it is frequently an interpretable design (effects on the outcome variable that are due to the treatment variable can be separated from effects due to extraneous variables), it is recommended when a true experimental design cannot be achieved (Cook & Campbell, 1979).

When the nonequivalent groups design is employed, the control group may also receive a treatment. The control group of patients might receive the traditional nursing intervention, whereas the experimental group would receive the innovative intervention being tested. This is true in the example of AD patient research. The two groups of subjects represent preexisting groups of patients who are separated from one another either temporally or spatially. With temporal separation, the two groups may represent different cohorts of patients who have received care at a single nursing service site. The control group could be patients who received care during the year prior to the institution of the innovative nursing intervention, whereas the treatment or experimental group could consist of patients who received care in the year following use of the innovative intervention. One example of spatial separation would be assigning patients on one patient care unit to the control group, where the traditional nursing care continues to be given, and assigning patients on another unit to the experimental group, which would receive the innovative intervention to be tested.

A study by Nath and Rinehart (1979) employed the nonequivalent group design to compare the effects of individual and group relaxation therapy on blood pressure of essential hypertensives. Fifteen hypertensives were taught progressive muscle relaxation. Nine were taught individually and six were taught as a group. The choice of individual or group instruction was made by the subjects. The relaxation teaching sessions were held once weekly for four weeks. Blood pressure measurements were taken at the beginning and end of each session, as well as at the beginning of the first and last sessions. No differences were found between the two methods of instruction. Decreases in both systolic and diastolic blood pressures from the beginning to the end of each session were found, as well as decreases in systolic pressure from the first session to the fourth. It was concluded (1) that group instruction and individual instruction are equally effective, (2) that progressive muscle relaxation is effective in reducing blood pressure, and (3) that four weeks is inadequate for reducing diastolic blood pressure.

Several threats to internal and external validity are associated with the basic nonequivalent group design. *Selection bias* is an especially relevant threat. It is important to distinguish two versions of the nonequivalent control group design. In one, two natural groups are available and the experimenter has free choice of who receives the treatment. In the other, the experimental group is self-selected and subjects deliberately seek out the treatment. In this case no control group is available from the same population. Selection interactions become more likely in the latter version.

In the Maas and Buckwalter research it was not possible to assign patients, staff, or family members randomly to experimental and control groups. Rather, patients were placed on the special care unit by agency admission procedures and according to the judgment of clinicians. The two groups of AD patients were likely to vary in their initial levels of functioning, falls, and medication use. Thus it is questionable whether any differences found after exposure to the special care unit are due to the treatment variable. Perhaps the patients who were not assigned to the special unit had a greater number of additional medical diagnoses that inhibited their functioning, or the experimental subjects might have been, on the average, more innately capable. To rule out such explanations, it is necessary to include assessments of other variables that may differ between the groups and that may affect the outcome variables. Statistical procedures such as analysis of covariance can then be employed to evaluate the viability of these alternative explanations.

The nonequivalent groups design is particularly vulnerable to the threat of *selection-maturation*. This occurs where one group has a preponderance of subjects who tire more easily or experience some other internal change that influences the criterion variable irrespective of the treatment effect. In the case of the evaluation of the special unit for AD patients, this type of threat is present if the two groups differ in the natural course of the Alzheimer's disease process. In this situation, effects attributed to the special unit may actually result from different patterns of naturally occurring changes in the disease over time for the two groups. One method that can be used to assist with the interpretation of this source of variation involves adding another measure of the criterion variable prior to exposure to the treatment being tested. Group mean differences can also be inspected to assess whether groups are maturing at different rates. If mean difference is due to selection only, the difference in growth between groups should also be occurring within groups. Thus one would expect an increase in within-group variances at posttest when compared to pretest (Cook & Campbell, 1979). Second, selection-maturation can be inferred from the regression of the maturation variable on the pretest outcome scores for both groups. Different linear slopes of the two regression lines indicate that there is a difference in the average change in the outcome scores in the two groups.

A problem may also arise due to the interaction of selection and history. Cook and Campbell (1979) refer to this threat to internal validity as *selection-history* or *local history*. These effects result from the combined influence of nonrandom selection of subjects and events that affect the groups differentially. *History* in this sense refers to any events occurring between the assessment periods that have an influence on the outcome variable(s). Events that affect one group more than the other are of particular concern. Therefore, the researcher carefully scrutinizes any events that may occur during the course of the study. An example of the threat of selection-history to the internal validity of the Alzheimer's study might be the exposure of subjects to programs, such as a friendly visitor program, that are extraneous to the study. If more subjects in one group are given the additional program or the program is given only to one group and it affects cognitive and functional abilities, it would be difficult to separate these effects from those of the special care unit program. Of course, these effects could serve to make the special care unit program appear more or less effective than it actually is. This would depend upon whether a greater percentage of experimental or control subjects were affected by the extraneous treatment program.

The remaining threats to internal validity that are relevant to the basic nonequivalent groups design have to do with measurement of the outcome variable(s). The first threat is *instrumentation*. This occurs when there are floor or ceiling effects, or when the units of measurement on a scale are not uniform. In other words, some scales are more or less sensitive to change at certain points on the scale than at other points. Inspection of the distribution of scores on the measure may indicate the presence of instrumentation problems. If so, the distributions will be skewed and/or the group means and variances will be correlated (Cook & Campbell, 1979). A potential instrumentation bias was discovered during pretest of the Family Perceptions Tool (Maas & Buckwalter, 1985) that was developed to measure the attitudes of family members regarding the care of their AD relatives. A possible ceiling effect occurred. The mean score of family members was 6.4 on a 7-point Likert-type scale, where 7 indicated the most positive attitude toward care the AD patient was receiving. This indicated that the instrument was not sensitive to variation in the attitudes of family members and that scores could not go above a certain level of positive attitude.

Regression is the final threat to internal validity that is relevant to the nonequivalent groups design. In this case, if the experimental AD group had much lower cognitive and functional abilities than the control group prior to the special unit intervention, the special unit would appear to be effective, in that the two groups do not appear to differ on the posttest measures. The change in cognitive and functional abilities scores could, however, be due to the measurement problem termed *regression toward the mean*. Due to errors in measurement, individuals who received extreme scores on an instrument at a first measurement are likely to receive scores closer to the population mean on that instrument at the second assessment. As a result, a group of individuals who receive extreme scores on a measure will tend to show a significant change on the measure at retesting toward the population mean in the absence of any real change in true scores. Thus the change in the experimental AD group could simply reflect regression toward the mean, and not indicate that the special unit program caused a significant improvement in cognitive and functional abilities.

In an effort to obtain groups whose scores are as equivalent as possible on pretest measures, researchers sometimes misguidedly match controls with experimental subjects known to have extreme scores. This results in the control group mean regressing to its population mean and the experimental group mean not regressing when the experimental subjects are not selected on the basis of their extreme scores. Obviously, true score comparisons are obscured in this circumstance.

One way of assessing the presence of regression artifacts is to employ multiple assessments prior to the intervention. This permits an evaluation of whether the differences reflect regression toward the mean or real treatment effects. The design for this Alzheimer's research project (Figure 3.1) contains multiple pretest measures and thus allows assessment of possible bias in the results due to statistical regression.

The *untreated control group design with pretest measures at more than one time interval* is the variation of the untreated control group design most commonly used (Cook & Campbell, 1979). This design is presented in Figure 3.3. There are advantages to administering pretests at more than one time that strengthen the basic nonequivalent groups design. Multiple pretests permit assessment of whether the groups are becoming disparate at different rates from O_1 to O_2, when the effect could not be due to the treatment (selection-maturation threat). Multiple pretests also allow assessment of spurious treatment effects due to statistical regression and provide an estimate of the correlation between O_2 and O_3 in the experimental group, as there was no exposure to the treatment, based on the $O_2 = O_3$ correlation in the control group. These correlations provide essential information for statistical analysis that will be discussed in more detail in a later section. Obviously, the correlation estimates are dependent on the test-retest interval, so it is best to maintain equal intervals between O_1 and O_2 and between O_2 and O_3.

$$O_1 \qquad O_2 \qquad X \qquad O_3$$

$$O_1 \qquad O_2 \qquad\qquad O_3$$

Figure 3.3. The Untreated Control Group Design with Pretest Measures at More Than One Time Interval
SOURCE: Cook and Campbell (1979). Reprinted by permission.
NOTE: See note to Figure 3.1 for explanation of figure elements.

Since the untreated control group with multiple pretests variation of the basic nonequivalent group design considerably strengthens the interpretation of results, it would seem that this quasi-experimental approach could be used more than it is. However, it is often problematic to obtain pretest measures when the field researcher is unable to delay implementation of the treatment. Furthermore, funding sources are often unwilling to expend monies for pretests, preferring instead to commit resources only for posttest measures. However, researchers should try to achieve the addition of at least one more pretest measure to the basic nonequivalent groups design, and should attempt to convince funding agencies of its merit for conducting quality studies.

Three additional variations of nonequivalent group designs are worthy of discussion because they can often be used by nurse researchers in field settings. These designs are useful when a nonequivalent control group cannot be obtained. These designs are applicable when the researcher must create circumstances that are conceptually similar to the no-treatment control group, or in other words, when only a single group of subjects is available for the research. The first of these designs, illustrated in Figure 3.4, is the *removed-treatment design with pretest and posttest*.

$$O_1 \quad X \quad O_2 \quad O_3 \quad \bar{X} \quad O_4$$

Figure 3.4. The Removed Treatment Design with Pretest and Posttest
SOURCE: Cook and Campbell (1979). Reprinted by permission.
NOTE: $\bar{X}$ = treatment removed; see note to Figure 3.1 for explanation of other elements.

Removed-Treatment Design with Pretest and Posttest

This design can be advantageous when subjects self-select out of a treatment. When the effects of interventions such as reminiscence therapy or exercise are being evaluated, patients often remove themselves from the intervention or are removed by factors that cannot be controlled. A single group pretest-posttest is fundamental. However, a third posttest is added, which is followed by removal of the treatment (X) and one more posttest. The O_3-O_4 data collections serve as the no-treatment control for the O_1-O_2 data collections. One group of subjects participates throughout the course of the study. When a treatment is effective, there are expected differences between O_1 and O_2 and between O_3 and O_4. These differences must be in opposite directions, with a clear change following removal of the treatment variable. This latter result is needed in order to distinguish differences between the experimental and control conditions that are due to removal of the treatment rather than to the treatment simply having no long-term effect.

One difficulty with this design is that in using it, it may be hard to demonstrate a pattern of effects upon which a valid statistical conclusion can be based. That is, the difference between O_1, O_2, and O_3, O_4, must not be equal, and the difference between O_2, O_3, and O_3, O_4, must also not be equal. Further, the researcher must be aware that maturation effects could explain any differences that occur. Another difficulty can arise with this design if the treatment has to be removed deliberately. Since the treatment was likely introduced because of its positive benefits, subjects may become frustrated and agitated when it is removed. These responses may correlate with the outcome measures and obscure the effect of the removed treatment. Thus the design may not be a good choice when the researcher must deliberately remove the treatment. Finally, it is important that observations be made at equal time intervals in order to assess any spontaneous changes that may be occurring with the passage of time, irrespective of the introduction and removal of the treatment.

The Repeated-Treatment Design

Figure 3.5 depicts the repeated-treatment design, in which the researcher uses a single group of subjects because he or she has access to only one population. Subjects are exposed to the treatment, removed from treatment, and then exposed again to the treatment. This design is best employed where the treatment effects are expected to dissipate rapidly or where the effects are expected to be cumulative. To interpret the effects of the treatment, the O_3, O_4, difference must be in the same direction as the O_1, O_2, difference. This design is vulnerable to regularly occurring extraneous sources of variance due to subject maturation or history. Further, there is potential for subject resentment or frustration when a treatment is removed, just as in the removed-treatment design with pretest and posttest, described above. This frustration can confound the O_3, O_4, difference, which could be inferred to be due to replication of the treatments when in fact it was due to a reduction in frustration when the treatment was again introduced. In order to enhance the external validity and statistical validity of the design, large samples of subjects should be used. The design is particularly vulnerable to the reactive effects of experimental procedures. Thus the design is best when the treatment being tested is unobtrusive and there is a long time interval before reintroduction of the treatment. In order to prevent the effects of extraneous cyclic rival causes, it is best to distribute reintroductions of the treatment randomly.

$$\text{O}_1 \quad \text{X} \quad \text{O}_2 \quad \bar{\text{X}} \quad \text{O}_3 \quad \text{X} \quad \text{O}_4$$

Figure 3.5. The Repeated Treatment Design
SOURCE: Cook and Campbell (1979). Reprinted by permission.
NOTE: See note to Figure 3.1 for explanation of figure elements.

The repeated-treatment design could be useful for testing many nursing interventions that are not especially conspicuous or invasive to the patient, such as interaction or psychosocial modalities, or touch or reflective techniques.

The Reversed-Treatment Nonequivalent Control Group Design with Pretest and Posttest

This design is diagrammed in Figure 3.6, where X+ represents an expected effect in one direction and X− represents an expected effect in the opposite direction (Cook & Campbell, 1979). The reversed-treatment design is resistant to selection-maturation threats because maturation rarely occurs at the same time in opposite directions in the two groups. It is also stronger than basic nonequivalent group designs in terms of construct validity because it necessitates a carefully specified causal theory in order to hypothesize an effect in one direction in one group and an opposite effect in the other group. Reactive effects of the experimental procedures are less likely to explain hypothesized effects that are obtained in many types of studies, because social desirability would be expected to ameliorate effects of the conceptually opposite treatment. However, this should not be taken to mean that the design is totally resistant to the Hawthorne effect. Cook and Campbell (1979) emphasize that to be maximally interpretable the reversed treatment design requires (1) a placebo control group that receives a treatment not expected to influence the outcome measure except through a reactive effect of experimental procedures, and (2) a control group that receives no treatment for a baseline of no cause.

The reversed-treatment design is often difficult to implement in social settings. Treatments that produce negative effects are considered

O_1	$X+$	O_2
O_1	$X-$	O_2

Figure 3.6. The Reversed Treatment Nonequivalent Control Group Design with Pretest and Posttest
SOURCE: Cook and Campbell (1979). Reprinted by permission.
NOTE: $X+$ and $X-$ = reversed treatments; see note to Figure 3.1 for explanation of other elements.

unethical. Thus the deliberate design of these experimental conditions is questionable. It may be possible, however, for nurse researchers to capture the reversed-treatment experimental conditions as natural, unplanned occurrences that result from changes in the availability of resources or differing philosophies regarding nursing administration, education, and practice.

The Cohort Design with Cyclical Turnover

The cohort design, Figure 3.7, can be useful for studies in which (1) some subjects (cohorts) are exposed to a treatment, as they cycle through an organization, while other subjects (cohorts) are not; (2) it can be assumed that the cohorts differ only minimally; and (3) archival records can be used to compare cohorts on specific characteristics. The extent to which groups can be assumed to be comparable depends upon the researcher's ability to examine background characteristics.

Hamera and O'Connell (1981) used this design to study the effects of primary and team nursing on patient-centered variables such as nurturance received, patient involvement, and frequency of nurse-patient contacts. Baseline observational data were collected on 12 randomly selected adult medical patients experiencing team nursing care. A primary nursing care approach was then implemented on the same nursing unit. Six months later, 12 randomly selected medical patients were observed under this system. Patients were observed 24 hours a day for five days of hospitalization. Results showed that there were no differences between primary and team nursing care groups in the number of contacts, nurturance, or patient involvement with all nursing personnel or with professional nurses. However, when the primary

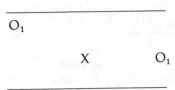

Figure 3.7. The Cohort Design with Cyclical Turnover
SOURCE: Cook and Campbell (1979). Reprinted by permission.
NOTE: See note to Figure 3.1 for explanation of figure elements.

group was adjusted to include only those patients for whom primary nursing care was fully implemented, the primary group received more nurturance and tended to be more actively involved than did the team group. *t*-tests indicated no statistically significant differences between the groups on age, number of days hospitalized, or number of patients observed over weekends, providing some check on selection bias. However, history could have differentially affected the groups during the 18-month span of the study. Further, the nursing personnel who implemented the two types of care may have been an extraneous source of variance due to characteristics and behavior that were not necessarily a function of the system of care. Unfortunately, the investigators did not report data for the nursing personnel who implemented team nursing and primary nursing.

INTERRUPTED TIME-SERIES DESIGNS

The basic interrupted time-series design involves multiple observations over time, usually with a single group of subjects. However, the time-series design can also use different but similar units of analysis (Cook & Campbell, 1979). Figure 3.8 depicts the basic interrupted time-series design. For nursing research, the design has particular relevance whenever a program or intervention is hypothesized to affect variables that are regularly measured and contained in archival sources. It is especially relevant for many quality assurance studies and also can be convenient for conducting "pure" research. Time-series analyses can supplement information gathered using nonequivalent group designs. This combination of methodologies represents a rigorous form of evaluation, even in the context of quasi-experimental design.

$$O_1 \quad O_2 \quad O_3 \quad O_4 \quad O_5 \quad X \quad O_6 \quad O_7 \quad O_8 \quad O_9 \quad O_{10}$$

Figure 3.8. Interrupted Time-Series Design
SOURCE: Cook and Campbell (1979). Reprinted by permission.
NOTE: See note to Figure 3.1 for explanation of figure elements.

In the Maas and Buckwalter (1985) Alzheimer's unit research example, two basic quasi-experimental designs (nonequivalent groups and time series) were combined. The combined design allowed the investigators to better interpret results that could potentially be confounded by the threats to internal validity that would be present if either of the two basic designs were used alone.

Time-series design variations become more complicated and combine a number of the nonequivalent group design variations. Combinations of variations provide the means whereby researchers can enhance their ability to interpret both of the basic quasi-experimental designs.

When the interrupted time-series design is used, the researcher must know exactly when the subjects were exposed to the treatment variable in order to infer its effects. If a treatment effect occurs, the outcome measures taken after exposure to the treatment should be different from those taken before exposure to the treatment. Hence the time-series measures are "interrupted."

At least 30 time periods should be available when the researcher considers using the interrupted time-series design. This allows sufficient data to be gathered for an evaluation of a trend over time following the intervention. Cook and Campbell (1979) describe several types of interruption effects that can occur. The first is a sharp change in mean scores when the interruption occurs, indicating different levels or intercepts of the slopes of pre- and posttreatment scores. The second interruption effect that can be observed is a change in the slope of the mean scores before and after treatment. In addition to changes in slope and intercept of mean scores, the interruption effect can also be characterized as continuous or discontinuous and as instantaneous or delayed. Note, however, that the different effects can occur simultaneously in various combinations.

A major strength of the basic time-series design is that it allows the assessment of outcome effects that are due to maturation prior to the introduction of a treatment. Multiple observations also make it possible to examine the trend of pretest scores for an effect that is due to statistical regression. Further, with a large number of time period observations, extraneous effects due to history or cyclic influences can also be evaluated. However, history remains the main threat to internal validity of the design. Data collections at frequent intervals (weekly versus monthly or yearly) and the careful recording of all possible events or circumstances that could reasonably influence outcomes should make it possible for the researcher to determine whether any event that occurred between the last pretest and the first posttest may have caused the interruption effect.

Instrumentation and selection bias are additional threats to the internal validity of the basic time-series design. Instrumentation can produce spurious effects due to differences in the way data are recorded or maintained over time. Changes can also come about in the way variables are conceptually and operationally defined. These sources of extraneous variance are most likely to result from changes in personnel or philosophy within an organization. However, they can also be the result of changes in the knowledge and motivation of key persons involved in the study. Selection effects threaten the validity of interpretation when changes in the experimental groups occur simultaneously with the introduction of the treatment. Often this occurs because the treatment itself causes subject attrition from the study. This problem can be resolved by restricting either all or part of the data analysis to a subset of the subjects from whom data on reliable and relevant background characteristics show a distinct change when the treatment is introduced. Selection is apt to be a problem if a distinct change is found.

Reactive effects of experimental procedures threaten the external validity of any study that uses a time-series design if the same subjects are measured at each time period and/or the subjects are aware of treatment exposure. These conditions are not likely to occur with archival studies, but they often exist with clinical nursing research, particularly when the time intervals are sufficiently short to make the recall of responses probable. The lack of availability of multiple measures of variables may also be a constraint when the researcher is dependent upon archival sources of data. Nurse administrators, researchers, nurses responsible for quality assurance studies, and clinical practitioners are advised to consider this potential constraint on the conduct of research prior to the collection of archival data.

Certainly the time-series design that has an adequate number of time period observations has a distinct advantage for generalization of results over a variety of time periods. A final advantage of the basic time-series design is the opportunity that is often present to examine results within subgroups of subjects. When this is possible the external validity of the design is strengthened. Subjects can be stratified according to individual and setting characteristics in order to determine if effects hold across subgroups. Of course, the researcher who uses archival data is limited to the variables measured in the setting and to the ranges of values recorded.

Interrupted Time-Series Designs with a Nonequivalent No-Treatment Group Time Series

The first variation on the basic interrupted time-series design results when a nonequivalent no-treatment group time series is added. This design is illustrated in Figure 3.9. This is the design used by Maas and Buckwalter (1985).

The addition of a no-treatment control group time series to the basic time-series design makes it strong in terms of the threat of history to internal validity because the effects of history can be tested. This design can still be subject to the threat of selection-history interaction, however, if one group is exposed to a unique event and the other is not. The threat can occur only if one group is influenced by an event *at the time that it is also exposed to the treatment*. The threat is enhanced by the addition of factors that increase the nonequivalence of the groups. These are viable threats for the Alzheimer's research example because one of the groups of subjects was housed on a unit that was

O_1	O_2	O_3	O_4	O_5	X	O_6	O_7	O_8	O_9	O_{10}
O_1	O_2	O_3	O_4	O_5		O_6	O_7	O_8	O_9	O_{10}

Figure 3.9. Interrupted Time-Series Design with a Nonequivalent No-Treatment Group Time Series
SOURCE: Cook and Campbell (1979). Reprinted by permission.
NOTE: See note to Figure 3.1 for explanation of figure elements.

O_{A1}	O_{A2}	O_{A3}	O_{A4}	O_{A5}	X	O_{A6}	O_{A7}	O_{A8}	O_{A9}	O_{A10}
O_{B1}	O_{B2}	O_{B3}	O_{B4}	O_{B5}		O_{B6}	O_{B7}	O_{B8}	O_{B9}	O_{B10}

Figure 3.10. The Interrupted Time Series with Nonequivalent Dependent Variables
SOURCE: Cook and Campbell (1979). Reprinted by permission.
NOTE: Letter subscripts = different measures; see note to Figure 3.1 for explanation of other elements.

isolated to some extent from the rest of the agency, and because subjects might have been selected for admission to the special care unit based on factors that made them noncomparable to control group subjects (e.g., more problem behaviors). Isolation from the other agency units could make the differential exposure of each of the groups to a unique situation even more likely.

The more comparable the groups are, the stronger this design is for testing other factors threatening the internal validity of the basic time-series design. Matching is not a solution for noncomparability. Rather, matching can produce the same distortion in the outcome due to regression effects as was described for the nonequivalent control group design. In general, the threats to external validity are the same as those described for the basic time-series design.

The Interrupted Time-Series Design with Nonequivalent Dependent Variables

This design, depicted in Figure 3.10, is included because of its value for testing the effects of history and for the advantage it has for enhancing construct validity. The effects of history can be assessed and the construct validity strengthened by collecting data for some variables that should show treatment effects and for others that should not.

For the nonequivalent dependent variables design, as well as for the interrupted time-series design with nonequivalent dependent variables, sufficient theory must exist to establish the conceptual relationship of the dependent variables. As with other designs, questions arise as to whether or not the relationships will hold for other populations and across subgroups of the target population.

Interrupted Time-Series Design
with Removed Treatment

Figure 3.11 illustrates this design, which is actually two interrupted time series joined together: O_1 to O_9 represents one time series that allows assessment of a treatment effect; O_5 to O_{13} allows assessment of the removal of the treatment.

For maximum inference of effect, the researcher would expect one form of change between O_4 and O_5 and an opposing change between O_9 and O_{10}. Certainly the design has all of the strengths characteristic of the simple time series. However, the second time series adds protection from the threat of history to internal validity. This is because any historical event that could pose a threat would have to operate in opposite directions at different times, or two events would have to operate in different directions at different times. Of course, the resentful demoralization described earlier in designs that remove subjects from treatment can also occur with this design. Thus the designs are best interpreted when the treatment is not perceived as particularly important to the subjects. Regardless of the effects of resentful demoralization, the design is quite strong because two alternative explanations are required in order to negate results that occur in a different direction after removal of a treatment.

$$O_1 \ O_2 \ O_3 \ O_4 \ O_5 \ X \ O_6 \ X \ O_7 \ X \ O_8 \ X \ O_9 \ X \ O_{10} \ O_{11} \ O_{12} \ O_{13}$$

Figure 3.11. Interrupted Time Series with Removed Treatment
SOURCE: Cook and Campbell (1979). Reprinted by permission.
NOTE: See note to Figure 3.1 for explanation of figure elements.

Interrupted Time-Series Design
with Switching Replications

In this design (Figure 3.12), two nonequivalent groups are exposed to a treatment and serve as control groups for each other. There are two important reasons for including this design in a discussion of quasi-experimentation. First, the design has strong internal and external validity. Second, it is a practical design that nurse researchers should consider whenever a nonequivalent control group is available. The ad-

O_1	O_2	O_3		O_4	O_5	O_6	O_7	O_8	X	O_9	O_{10}	O_{11}
O_1	O_2	O_3	X	O_4	O_5	O_6	O_7	O_8		O_9	O_{10}	O_{11}

Figure 3.12. Interrupted Time Series with Switching Replications
SOURCE: Cook and Campbell (1979). Reprinted by permission.
NOTE: See note to Figure 3.1 for explanation of figure elements.

vantage of replication built into the design makes it possible to extend the findings beyond a single population. In view of the considerable costs of conducting research studies, this efficiency should be most attractive. Furthermore, one should expect that cooperating settings, from which nonequivalent control groups are obtained, would find the demonstration of treatment effects in these groups beneficial. An additional advantage for nursing is the potential for greater utilization of findings by settings where effects of a treatment have been demonstrated, causing them to acquire a more vested interest in the research. One additional benefit of the switching replications time-series design is that it makes it possible to assess delayed effects. If the effect is delayed equally in each group, it should be observed in an earlier discontinuity in one group.

Interrupted Time-Series Design with Multiple Replications

The interrupted time-series design is presented in Figure 3.13. The design is very powerful for testing causal hypotheses, and has the added advantage of modifications that allow the testing of more than one treatment in a single study, as well as interaction effects of treatments. Two treatments can be tested by substituting X_1 for X and X_2 for X.

Parsons, Smith-Peard, and Page (1985) used the interrupted time-series design with multiple replications to assess the effects of oral, body, and catheter care on the cerebrovascular status of 19 severe closed head injured patients. Measures of heart rate, arterial blood pressures, intracranial pressures, and cerebral perfusion pressures were taken at baseline, peak nursing intervention, and one-minute recovery times for each patient. Statistically significant increases in the dependent variables were observed at peak intervention. By recovery time these

$$O_1 \quad O_2 \ X \ O_3 \quad O_4 \ \bar{X} O_5 \quad O_6 \ X \ O_7 \quad O_8 \ \bar{X} O_9 \quad O_{10} \ X \ O_{11} \quad O_{12} \ X \ O_{13} \quad O_{14}$$

Figure 3.13. Interrupted Time Series with Multiple Replications
SOURCE: Cook and Campbell (1979). Reprinted by permission.
NOTE: $\bar{X}$ = treatment removed; see note to Figure 3.1 for explanation of other elements.

values had returned to baseline levels. Since cerebral perfusion pressures never fell below 50 mm Hg., the three hygiene interventions were considered safe for the patient with closed head injury.

Martinson and Anderson (1983) used another variation of the interrupted time-series design with multiple replications to study the effects of thermal applications to the abdomens of four dogs. A silicone rubber envelope through which water circulated at 0, 10, 20, 30, 40, or 50 degrees centigrade was applied. Skin surface, subcutaneous, intraperitoneal, intestinal, and colonic temperatures were measured at baseline (10 minutes after starting the procedure) and 90 minutes after application of the thermal pad. For the control conditions (no pad) measurements were taken at 10 minutes and 100 minutes after initiation of the procedure. The first 100-minute procedure for each dog was a no-pad treatment. Then, the 6 thermal applications were chosen at random without replacement. The eighth 100-minute procedure was another no-pad treatment. This was followed by 6 additional random thermal applications, 1 no-pad treatment, 6 thermal applications, 1 no-pad treatment, 6 thermal, and 1 final no-pad treatment. Each dog had 24 sessions of temperature application and 6 sessions of no-pad application. Results of the study showed that both cutaneous and subcutaneous temperatures were affected by surface application of heat and cold to the area, while core temperature remained unaffected.

As with the removed treatment design (Figure 3.11), the direction of treatment and removal of treatment must be opposite. Further, a treatment effect can be inferred if the same pattern of effects for both the treatment and its removal occurs throughout the data collection. The design is vulnerable to the extraneous effects of cyclical maturation, so random scheduling of treatments and their removal is suggested, while preserving the alternating treatment and removal, unless cyclic effects can be ruled out by a strong theoretical base.

Practicality is, however, a weakness of this design. The design is possible only when the effects of a treatment are expected to extinguish rapidly. Also, the design ordinarily requires that the researcher have the ability to control the circumstances of the experiment. This is usually not possible with nursing phenomena, although educational and mental health settings may be exceptions. For example, it may be a useful design for testing forms of behavior modification interventions.

In conclusion, a number of problems may arise with time-series designs that have not been included in the discussion thus far. First, some treatments cannot be introduced quickly—rather, their impact on subjects evolves over time. Second, treatment effects may have a variety of periods of delay that differ among specific populations and from one time to another. Third, although an abundance of archival data exist that theoretically could be used for time-series analysis, they are often difficult to locate and the researcher may have problems obtaining their release. The time intervals of archival data may also be inappropriate for the research. Data may be missing or unreliable. Fourth, it is often problematic to obtain the 30 or more observations recommended for data analysis. Because of the advantages of these designs for nursing research and the problems that have just been listed, nurse administrators, educators, researchers, and clinicians are encouraged to consider their potential applications and to anticipate their use when data are routinely gathered and stored. Many of these designs could be employed with relative ease to answer nursing questions if these recommendations are followed.

ISSUES OF DATA ANALYSIS
FOR NONEQUIVALENT GROUP DESIGNS

Data analysis for quasi-experimental designs presents a number of complex problems. With nonequivalent group designs, pretreatment differences between the experimental and control groups on the outcome variables are often present due to the nonrandom selection process and other sources of extraneous variance discussed above. Because these pretest differences may produce posttest differences even without a treatment effect, the analysis must *control* for the effects of the initial differences. In other words, to evaluate whether the treatment produced a significant difference between the experimental and control groups, it is necessary to equate the two groups of subjects.

There are several statistical procedures that can be used to separate the effect of the treatment from the effects of other variable threats to the internal validity of the relationship under study. Analysis of variance (ANOVA), analysis of covariance (ANCOVA), analysis of variance with blocking or matching, and analysis of variance with gain scores are four of the more common procedures (Reichardt, 1979). Each of these procedures is appropriate under specific conditions for the analysis of nonequivalent group designs; the four procedures should not be used interchangeably.

Analysis of Variance

Analysis of variance is the simplest, but least powerful, of the four procedures. ANOVA provides three components of the structure of the data: (1) the grand mean of the posttest scores, the average response on the measurement scale; (2) the treatment effect, the average value that the treatment adds to or subtracts from the posttest scores in the treatment group; and (3) the error (residual), the value that represents all extraneous factors contributing to differences between the scores. Pretest scores are not assessed in this model, nor are interaction treatment effects. Further, ANOVA explains only the proportion of variance in the posttest scores that is due to the treatment, and assigns all other variation to the error term. The treatment is assumed to be the single cause of the posttest difference between the experimental and control groups. Though ANOVA can be used to assess differences between groups on the pretest, and though this may be better than ignoring the pretest differences altogether, assuming the groups to be equivalent based on "no significant difference" in pretest scores will likely lead to biased results. This is because the procedure cannot assess variation due to such factors as selection-maturation. Although the groups are equivalent based on their pretest scores, they can become different over time due to the interaction of selection and maturation. Thus the ANOVA on the posttest could result in a statistically significant but spurious difference.

Analysis of Covariance

A statistical procedure that can be used to equate the two groups is analysis of covariance. When pretreatment differences are present between the experimental and control groups, it cannot be automatically concluded that the posttreatment differences reflect the effects of the treatment. However, use of the pretreatment measure as a covariate can serve to equate the two groups on the outcome variable measure prior to the treatment, and thus isolate the effects of the treatment variable.

One problem with the use of ANCOVA to analyze data from a quasi-experimental design is that the statistical procedure is affected by errors of measurement in the covariate. Thus error in the covariate results in an underestimate for group differences on the pretreatment measure, and equates the treatment and control groups only if the covariate is error free (i.e., has a reliability of 1.00) (Reichardt, 1979). The issue of measurement error can also undermine attempts to equate groups by using other variables as covariates.

The LISREL program developed by Joreskog and Sorbom (1984) provides an approach for solving this problem. The program was designed to permit testing of theoretical models involving relationships among latent or unobserved variables. Scores on these latent variables are estimated by employing a number of measured variables that are designed to assess the construct represented by the latent variables. For example, a latent variable representing the functional ability of Alzheimer's patients in the LISREL procedure would be estimated by employing a number of different indicators (preferably three or more) (Bentler, 1980). The procedure is designed to derive a true score for subjects on the constructs being assessed that is uncontaminated by measurement error. Therefore, LISREL could be used to conduct an analysis of covariance where the biasing effects of measurement error in the covariate are eliminated.

Analysis of Variance with Blocking or Matching

There are advantages to using blocking or matching over ANOVA or ANCOVA. The block design adds a test for whether there is interaction of selection with the treatment. In nonequivalent group designs, subjects are blocked or matched on their pretest scores after they have been selected for experimental and control groups. Bias is a problem with this procedure due to the likelihood of imperfect matching. With blocking, effectiveness increases and approaches that of ANCOVA the greater the number of blocks that are used.

Analysis of Variance with Gain Scores

An analysis of variance using gain scores examines the change that occurs from pretest to posttest scores (Reichardt, 1979). The gain scores (posttest minus pretest) are used as the dependent variable for the ANOVA procedure. This approach assumes that a treatment effect would result in more or less change in the experimental group than in the control group. The analysis of variance with gain scores does not allow an assessment of interaction of the treatment with pretest. As with the ANCOVA procedure, additional variables can be added to the gain score analysis. However, gain score analysis should be used with caution, since the procedure cannot assess selection-maturation, instrumentation (floor and ceiling effects), or statistical regression effects.

To summarize, statistical procedures such as analysis of variance and covariance are appropriate for randomized designs. However, for quasi-experimental designs, there are problems associated with employing analysis of variance and covariance analyses. The LISREL procedure has promise for overcoming the biasing effects of measurement error in covariance analyses, and in permitting a more appropriate and powerful analysis of data from quasi-experimental designs. Most important, however, the statistical procedure used must be carefully selected to fit the particular characteristics of the data to be analyzed.

ISSUES OF DATA ANALYSIS WITH TIME-SERIES DESIGNS

Analysis with time-series designs uses statistical significance to affirm and bear out the magnitude of change that is observed with the naked eye when subjects are exposed to a treatment. However, the researcher should not be overly dependent upon these procedures. Certainly they are important, but they do not in themselves provide sufficient evidence of a treatment effect.

Statistical procedures based on ordinary least squares analysis are not appropriate for time-series data analysis (McCain & McCleary, 1979), principally because ordinary least squares assume independent errors and with any time-series design the errors are serially related (autocorrelated). This results in biased standard deviations of the estimates of parameters, as well as biased significance tests.

Autoregressive integrated moving average (ARIMA) models and the modeling techniques developed by Box and Jenkins (1976) are recommended for analysis of time-series data (McCain & McCleary, 1979).

These procedures estimate the systematic portion of the autocorrelation among time-series scores so that unbiased estimates of standard deviations can be calculated for the statistical tests. While the ARIMA procedures are less familiar to researchers who employ time-series designs, they should be used in preference to ordinary least squares tests. Experience with visual interpretation of time-series data according to specific principles is especially recommended with statistical tests used only to corroborate visual analysis.

SUMMARY

Quasi-experimental designs offer a variety of alternative strategies for the conduct of nursing field research. They are especially important for assessing causal relationships between nursing interventions and desired patient outcomes when the researcher is unable to implement all of the characteristics of a true experimental design. Although quasi-experimental designs are not as elegant for the control of threats to internal validity, and are therefore not as rigorous as true experimental designs for testing causal relationships, the nurse researcher who is knowledgeable about the variety of quasi-experimental designs can often combine the strengths of nonequivalent groups and time-series designs to optimize controls on internal validity. A substantial increase in the number of clinical nursing field studies conducted with many different populations could result, which would have the additional advantage of improving generalizability of findings.

REFERENCES

Bentler, P. M. (1980). Multivariate analysis with latent variables: Causal modeling. *Annual Review of Psychology, 31*, 419-456.

Box, G. E. P., & Jenkins, G. M. (1976). *Time series analysis: Forecasting and control.* San Francisco: Holden-Day.

Brink, P. J., & Wood, M. J. (1983). *Basic steps in planning nursing research: From question to proposal* (2nd ed.). Monterey, CA: Wadsworth Health Sciences.

Campbell, D. T., & Stanley, J. C. (1963). *Experimental and quasi-experimental designs for research.* Chicago: Rand McNally.

Cook, T. D., & Campbell, D. T. (Eds.) (1979). *Quasi-experimentation: Design and analysis issues for field settings.* Chicago: Rand McNally.

Hamera, E., & O'Connell, K. A. (1981). Patient-centered variables in primary and team nursing. *Research in Nursing and Health, 4*(1), 183-192.

Joreskog, R. G., & Sorbom, D. (1984). *LISREL: Analysis of linear structural relationships by the methods of maximum likelihood (version VI)*. Mooresville, IN: Software.

Maas, M. L., & Buckwalter, K. C. (1985). *Evaluation of a special Alzheimer's unit*. Proposal submitted to the American Nurses Foundation, Kansas City, MO.

Martinson, I. M., & Anderson, S. E. (1983). Effects of thermal applications on the abdominal temperature of dogs. *Research in Nursing and Health, 6*(2), 89-94.

McCain, L. J., & McCleary, R. (1979). The statistical analysis of the simple interrupted time-series quasi-experiment. In T. D. Cook & D. T. Campbell (Eds.), *Quasi-experimentation: Design and analysis issues for field settings*. Chicago, Rand McNally.

Nath, C., & Rinehart, J. (1979). Effects of individual and group relaxation therapy on blood pressure in essential hypertensives. *Research in Nursing and Health, 2*(3), 119-126.

Parsons, L. C., Smith-Peard, A. L., & Page, M. C. (1985). The effects of hygiene interventions on the cerebrovascular status of severe closed head injured persons. *Research in Nursing and Health, 8*(2), 173-182.

Reichardt, C. S. (1979). The statistical analysis of data from nonequivalent group designs. In T. D. Cook & D. T. Campbell (Eds.), *Quasi-experimentation: Design and analysis issues for field settings*. Chicago: Rand McNally.

PART III
SURVEY DESIGNS

All survey designs specify the relationship of two or more variables without any experimental manipulation of the independent variable. These designs do not control the independent variable and therefore do not have sufficient *internal validity* to support a cause-and-effect relationship. The strength of these designs lies in their *external validity*. They provide the means of examining variables within random samples of target populations and of drawing conclusions about the target populations from the sample data. Since no manipulation of variables occurs in these designs, they provide information about naturally occurring phenomena in a way that is not possible in experimental designs. Survey designs always incorporate statistical analysis of the relationships between and among variables in order to draw conclusions from the data.

In the case of the comparative survey, the dependent variable is measured and compared across groups, while the independent variable is simply observed as it occurs naturally in the population. The comparative design is theory based, as is the experimental design, and research findings derived through this design can be used to strengthen theory. Since, however, the design does not allow the independent variable to be manipulated, it cannot be used to test theory directly. Even when the most sophisticated statistical analysis is applied to data and used to test a predictive hypothesis, the lack of investigator control over the independent variable limits internal validity. The question to be answered using the comparative design is different from that of the experimental design: What are the differences between groups when the groups represent different positions of the independent variable and why does this difference result? A theoretical framework is used to predict cause and effect, although both the independent and dependent variables are observed as they occur naturally in the environment without investigator interference. These studies are frequently considered preliminary to the experimental design, as a beginning test of theory prior to actual experimentation.

The comparative design is the design of choice when it is either unethical or impossible to manipulate the independent variable. Studies comparing ethnic groups, age cohorts, and people with particular pathologies are all necessarily comparative rather than experimental. In a comparative design, however, such variables must be proposed as independent causative variables with predictive directional hypotheses of the anticipated results. Again, the significant difference between the comparative and experimental design is that in the comparative design the independent variable is *not* manipulated by the researcher.

In the correlational survey, two or more variables are measured as they exist in the population and their relationship is analyzed. Even when one of the variables is known to occur first in time, its effect on the dependent variable may not be predicted with any certainty. The initial question asked is, What is the relationship between or among these variables? The answer is a statistical description of the relationships. The design is supported by a conceptual framework. Although correlational surveys vary greatly in the strength of the framework, they must include potential explanations for the possible relationships among the variables. These explanations are derived from previous exploratory or descriptive studies or from theoretical propositions.

The comparative survey design exerts less control over the independent variable than does the quasi-experimental design, but more control than does the correlational survey. The correlational design is frequently used when there is limited knowledge of which variables in the design are independent and which are dependent, whereas in the comparative design the independent variable is used as the basis for formulating the groups. For both types of survey designs, the critical issue is external validity, and for maximum effectiveness, both require large, representative samples of the population. Accuracy of measurement is also critical, with measurement assumed to be primarily at the numeric level. Both designs are inherently descriptive and not directly theory testing, although they have both been used by researchers to test and to generate theory.

4. Comparative Designs

Marilynn J. Wood
Pamela J. Brink

Comparative designs can be many things, but they all have at least one thing in common—two or more groups are compared on some criterion. This chapter focuses on a special comparative design in which the groups are chosen because they represent different positions of an independent variable that we are interested in testing. We recognize that there are a variety of "comparative" designs that do not meet the specifications set forth in this chapter, but we feel strongly that the design described here can be used as a model, and that other comparative designs can be evaluated according to how well they meet these criteria.

We call this design the *comparative survey design*, and it is used instead of an experimental design when the theory base for the study meets the criteria for an experimental design (i.e., hypotheses could be tested) but for some reason the investigator cannot manipulate the independent variable and therefore cannot do an experiment. To use this design, it must be possible to find already-existing groups that differ on the independent variable. We can predict how the dependent variable should vary among these groups. Let us say that we are interested in a particular concept (such as social support) and wonder if specific patient outcomes will vary according to this characteristic. Since we cannot manipulate the characteristic, and since there has been a good deal of research on that characteristic, we eliminate both the experimental and the exploratory designs as designs of choice. Our decision, then, lies somewhere in the range of survey designs, comparative or correlational. Because prior research has shown a relationship between the characteristic and other variables in a particular population, we can now refine our study of that variable by discriminating among groups that differ on this characteristic. In so doing, we move from a correlational design to a comparative design in which we look for group differences on relevant dependent variables, having set up the groups to represent different positions of the independent variable—in this case, social support. Two or more groups would be identified for this study based upon their level of social support. In addition, because of the extent of theoretical knowledge we have about social support, we can develop hypotheses to predict the outcome for each group. This design allows theory testing without manipulation of the independent variable, but of course the results must be properly interpreted in light of the design's shortcomings compared to a true experiment.

Two basic situations arise in which the independent variable cannot be deliberately manipulated: (a) when an ethically unacceptable outcome would result from the manipulation, such as creating a toxic condition in the subjects, or (b) when the variable is a trait or characteristic of the subject that cannot be changed, such as age, ethnicity, or place of birth. In these instances, a comparative survey design allows the researcher to look at the effects of an independent variable on a dependent variable without direct intervention or manipulation of the independent variable. Two features of this design are critical. First, since random assignment is not possible, the groups must be comparable on the major extraneous variables, ideally differing only in the independent variable. In addition, because the design allows the researcher to predict the effect of the independent variable on the dependent variable, it is essential to have a theoretical farmework that explains the cause-and-effect relationship between these variables.

The comparative design is primarily utilized in field studies. Observations are made in naturalistic environments rather than in controlled laboratory settings in order to observe cause-and-effect relationships without manipulation or other interference. The design, however, can also be used as a field test prior to the development of an experiment.

BASIC OR CLASSICAL DESIGN

This is a two-group (treatment and contrast) design, similar to the basic experimental design, except that the two groups already exist.

The treatment group has the independent variable and the contrast group does not. A posttest measures only the dependent variable(s), which should yield interval- or ratio-level data. The study will usually be prospective, because the sample is selected based upon the independent variable. The classic example of this design can be found in the studies on smoking and lung cancer. As ealy as 1950, correlational designs established an association between these two variables. Since that time, many comparative studies have been done using smokers and nonsmokers. In some studies, smokers have been divided into groups based on sex, age, and smoking patterns such as duration of smoking and number of cigarettes smoked per day (the independent variables). The dependent variable was onset of lung cancer. More recent research has considered the work environment of the smoker as a possible independent variable to determine whether there are certain other persistent daily factors that contribute to the onset and type of lung cancer (U.S. DHHS, 1982).

Variations on the Basic Design

Many variations on the basic comparative design can be found. Comparative designs can use multiple groups differentiated on the independent variable. For instance, several types of nurse management systems can be compared on one or more patient outcome measures. Comparative designs can use time-series measurements of the dependent variable. If the study uses available data, such as a chart review, time-series measurements (multiple measures of the dependent variable over time) can occur both before and after the occurrence of the independent variable. Comparative studies can be retrospective if the sample is chosen on the basis of the dependent variable rather than the independent variable. Some studies of smoking and lung cancer are currently being conducted as retrospective studies, with the three types of lung cancer, as ascertained by microscopic examination, being traced back (retrospectively) to amount and type of smoking, age of smoking onset, sex, and work environment (U.S. DHHS, 1982).

Basic Assumptions of Comparative Designs

The following are the assumptions implicit in comparative designs:

(1) One can build support for cause and effect without the manipulation of the independent variable.

(2) There is enough knowlege about the variable(s) to develop predictive hypotheses based upon theory and prior research.
(3) One can establish comparable groups using sampling methodology.
(4) External validity can be achieved by utilizing a sample that is representative of the population.
(5) Measurement of the dependent variable will be accurate.
(6) Sampling and data analysis methods will control for extraneous variables so that the difference(s) between or among groups on the dependent variable can be identified.

CONTROL OVER DATA

The data in comparative designs are controlled through sample selection methods, by the conditions under which the independent and dependent variables are measured, and by the statistical techniques used to analyze the data. There is no manipulation of the independent variable because it has already occurred; therefore the action of the independent variable is observed rather than controlled. Instead, the independent variable is controlled through sample selection. The investigator selects the sample so that it is possible to discriminate between and among groups on the basis of the presence, absence, or amount of the independent variable. All relevant extraneous variables are measured so that their effect on the dependent variable can be estimated.

SAMPLES

A large simple random sample of the population is the ideal and should provide a representative sample from which comparison groups can be formulated unless one or more of the subgroups is expected to be proportionately small. In these cases, stratified random samples are the ideal and are used whenever population parameters are known. The sample is stratified on the independent variable by examining the available population (frequently through census records). The strata are developed and the percentage of the population within each stratum is noted. The sample can have the same proportions as in the population, but at times it may be advisable to have equal numbers from each stratum. Computing sample size from the available population is based upon the decision regarding the amount of sampling error allowable for the study. Stratified random samples ensure external validity (generalizability) of the results.

Sample Variations

When the total available population is small, or when the population parameters are unknown, quota samples may be drawn based upon the independent variable. These quota samples may sometimes be proportionate to the total population, or sometimes groups of equal size are used. Another sample variation is seen in the use of convenience samples that can be found to exist representing the various positions of the independent variable. For example, in a study of stress in ICU versus non-ICU nurses, the staff of the intensive care units was compared to the staff of general medical-surgical units to see if there was a significant difference in their levels of stress (Keane, Ducette, & Adler, 1985). Comparative designs may also be used to compare total populations to similar total populations. This is common in anthropological research, in which individual populations are studied independently using the single case descriptive design. The available data obtained through ethnography are then used for secondary analysis in a comparative design. On the assumption that the comparative analysis of single cases builds anthropological theory about human groups, the Human Relations Area Files (HRAF) were developed at Harvard for the sole purpose of providing a data base to use in comparing anthropological studies of culture groups. Because human groups cannot be manipulated easily (or, perhaps, ethically), the HRAF provide a needed data set for comparative analysis. Major universities throughout the United States have either complete or partial HRAF in the original paper format or on microfiche.

Another variation on sample selection involves drawing the random sample from two different populations, such as the runners and nonrunners used in the Walsh study reported below. Although the samples represented their respective populations (runners and students), they did not constitute a representative sample of the desired target population, and the results must therefore be viewed with caution.

The issues that need to be addressed in sample selection procedures are that the sample is representative of the population and that the comparison groups are equivalent on all relevant variables except the independent variable.

METHODS OF DATA COLLECTION

Any method of data collection is acceptable: observation, interview, questionnaire, projective tests, physiological tests, available data. The type of measurement will vary according to the questions asked, the hypotheses being tested, and the situation within which the study is to be conducted. The reliability and validity of the instruments are critical in this design because validity of the results will depend on accurate discrimination among groups. The best or preferred type of measurement is quantitative, using interval and ratio scales in order to use parametric statistics. Nominal and ordinal scales are used frequently and are quite acceptable so long as they are numerical rather than qualitative.

Possible sources of error in data collection procedures include the possibility of acquiescent response set in interviews, response bias in both interviews and questionnaires, and the Hawthorne effect among subjects in all comparative studies. Inaccurate transcription of data onto data collection forms or misinterpretation of meaning in written documentation are also possible sources of error in this design, as in all research.

RELIABILITY AND VALIDITY OF MEASUREMENT

In comparative studies, as with experimental designs, the critical issue is determining whether or not the groups differ with regard to the dependent variable. The accuracy of the measurement technique, therefore, becomes paramount. All measurement tools must have at least content validity—that is, they must be based upon the known literature on the topic. However, the quality of the study really depends on the quality of measurement, and therefore the use of well-tested instruments is recommended. Because this level of research is built upon theory and the findings of previous studies, it is not advisable to proceed without well-developed instruments. The subsequent results would not reflect the desired results in terms of hypothesis testing. The researcher must be able to rely upon the measurement tool to measure the dependent variable accurately. Therefore, norm-referenced or criterion-referenced validity of measurement tools is extremely important. Reliablity of the instruments must be estimated for the study population. Remember that reliability estimates are not a stable property of an instrument, but are specific to the use of that instrument with a particular population under specific measurement conditions (Cronbach, 1970; Lynn, 1985; Nunnally, 1978).

DATA ANALYSIS

The basic question asked by this design is, What are the differences between/among groups on the dependent variable? Assuming probability sampling techniques and interval/ratio levels of measurement, the test of choice in a two group design is the *t*-test. The *t*-test compares the means of two groups and examines the probability of getting this magnitude of difference by chance alone. It is particularly useful in designs requiring the comparison of two groups.

If there are multiple groups based on a categorical independent variable, the quantitative measures of the dependent variable, a one-way analysis of variance (ANOVA) is appropriate. ANOVA tells us whether the group means differ from one another. It assumes that the independent variable is at the nominal level. A "one-way" ANOVA indicates that there is only one independent variable. (ANOVA can also be used with multiple independent variables.) The dependent variable is assumed to be measured on an interval or ratio scale.

Quite commonly in comparative surveys, however, the comparative groups will be based on a quantitative independent variable, such as level of income or preoperative stress level, and a quantitative dependent variable that may or may not be measured at the interval level. In these cases, the appropriate test will be regression analysis (see Chapter 5 for further discussion of this technique).

Covariance analysis is a useful procedure in comparative as well as experimental designs for statistically removing differences among the comparison groups when they are not equivalent on significant ex-

traneous variables. Through the use of this technique, a statistical control can sometimes be provided for extraneous variables when direct
control through experimental design is impossible. The error variance
is reduced by controlling for variation in the dependent measure that
comes from separate measurable variables that influence all the group-
ings being compared (Munro, Visintainer, & Page, 1986, p. 218).
Analysis of covariance (ANCOVA) is a special case of the linear model.
Regression analysis is usually used in survey designs, and analysis of
variance in experimental designs. Wildt and Ahtola (1978) explain
analysis of covariance as a combination of these two techniques.
Therefore, an understanding of these two techniques is expected when
discussing covariance. The usual problem in comparative surveys
comes when the investigator is interested in the effect of an independent variable, either quantitative or categorical, on a quantitative dependent variable, but one or more "nuisance" variables (covariates) are
influencing the dependent variable in a linear fashion. Covariance
analysis first removes the effects of the covariates and then examines
the relationship between the independent and dependent variable. As
with ANOVA, it is assumed that the independent variable is nominal,
the dependent variable is continuous, and the covariates are measured
at the interval or ratio level. It is also assumed that a covariate has a
linear relationship with the dependent variable. If this assumption is
violated, the results will be of little value.

Take, for example, a study examining the differences between two
techniques of pain management used in two different clinical areas.
In a comparative design, the two techniques and their effect on the
level of pain perceived by the recipients would be observed as they
occur, since no manipulation of treatmens would be controlled by the
researcher. In this case, individual differences in the subjects might
influence their response to the treatment. These differences are then
identified as age and prior experience with surgery. By measuring age
and prior experience, and treating them as covariates, the researcher
is able to adjust for the differences in the subjects' level of perceived
pain that might be related to these two nuisance variables, thus providing a more accurate assessment of the effect of the two treatments.
This approach would remove any bias that might occur because the
two groups were not matched on these variables.

CRITIQUE

The first step in critiquing a comparative study is to evaluate whether it sets out to study "differences between and among groups." The next critical step is to determine whether the sample selection technique meets the basic assumptions of the design. A third consideration is the accuracy of the measurement techniques: To what extent are the issues of reliability and validity addressed? Fourth, one must judge whether the data analysis is appropriate to the question asked. Are the limitations of the design recognized? Finally, one must consider whether the findings are interpreted in light of the question asked and in terms of the limitations.

Another important issue in the critique of comparative designs is that of sources of error that might have come from data collection, sample selection, or choice of statistical test, as well as from transcription and coding of data. Each of these sources of error will affect the outcome of the study. The answer to the question, What are the differences between (or among) the groups (or measurements)? should have been accurately predicted by the theoretical framework. If the answer to the question does not support the predictive hypotheses, one should look first for weaknesses in the theory, then for decision errors in sampling, methods, and analysis of data. If the results do support the predictive hypotheses, the author's interpretation of the findings in light of the theoretical framework should be examined. This design cannot be expected to have strong internal validity, and therefore the interpretation of the findings should reflect this limitation.

ETHICAL ISSUES

A major concern with comparative designs is the protection of the anonymity of the groups used for comparisons. Identifying data must be obscured in the final report. When using total populations, each member of the total population must be given the right to refuse to participate even though replacement is not possible in this instance. Another issue that can arise in comparative designs comes from the possibility of serious weaknesses in the design that might negate any findings. In this case, it may be unethical to ask subjects to participate when there is no possibility of the study producing valid results. Finally, if the study examines a sensitive topic, subjects may need assistance in coping with the findings. If this is the case, subjects should be informed of resources for follow-up support.

EXAMPLES FROM THE LITERATURE

Laffrey (1986) examined perceived weight, perceived health status, health conception, and health behavior choices in normal-weight and overweight adults. Three research questions were addressed:

(1) Do perceived weight, perceived health status, health conception, and health behavior choice differ between normal-weight and overweight adults?
(2) What are the relationships among perceived health status, health conception, and health behavior choice in normal-weight adults?
(3) What are the relationships among perceived health status, health conception, and health behavior choice in overweight adults?

A random sample of 59 households in a midwestern suburban community produced 33 normal-weight and 26 overweight adults (25 men and 34 women). All subjects were white and had been born in the United States; ages ranged from 19 to 66 (mean age was 39 for normoweights, 43 for overweights). All overweights were at least 10-20% over the normal weight for their height (two were over 20% above normal weight). Education ranged from 5 to 18 years of school (mean 13.5 for normoweights and 13.7 for overweights). The two groups were similar on marital status and reported religion. Family income was lower in the normal weight group ($29,000 versus $35,000 for the overweight group).

Perceived weight was measured by asking the subjects to rate themselves as underweight, normal, or overweight. This response was validated by also asking them to compare themselves with others of their gender and age on a 3-point scale: weight less than others, weight same as others, or weight more than others. Perceived health status (PHS) was measured using a Cantril ladder, ranging from 1 (worst health I can imagine) to 10 (best health I can imagine).

Health conception measure (HCM) was a 16-item tool developed for this study. Content validity and a test-retest reliability coefficient of .76 after one week were reported. Health behavior choice scale (HBCS) was a 15-item tool to measure the reasons an individual chooses to engage in five health behaviors. Content validity and test-retest reliability coefficient of .93 were reported for this tool.

Body weight was measured using a GE portable digital scale. Subjects were asked their height without shoes and were measured if unsure. Weight-height ratios were compared with the norms of the Michigan Department of Public Health to establish normoweight versus overweight groups.

A *t*-test analysis of the differences between group means demonstrated no significant differences between the two groups on perceived health status, health conception, or health behavior choice. In addition, health conception and health behavior choice were significantly correlated in both groups. The relationship between perceived health status and health conception was positive and significant only in the normoweight group. No other significant relationships were found.

There are two major problems with this study: the weakness of the conceptual framework and the sample size. The author did not distinguish between "overweight" and "obesity" as health hazards, yet the literature states that between 50% and 100% over "normal" weight to height ratios is required before there is any significant difference in health hazard. Therefore, individuals between 10% and 20% overweight are not "at risk" in the epidemiological sense. The prediction that individuals not at risk would perceive themselves to be at risk was somewhat weak. Second, the size of the "overweight" group (26 individuals, with only 2 over 20% overweight) was simply too small to make any predictions about overweight or "obese" subjects. Finally, the literature is very clear that American women generally tend to perceive themselves as overweight even when they are of normal weight, so perceived weight for women will be skewed in that direction, regardless of actual weight. The author is to be commended for attempting a random sample, but some populations are so difficult to find that random samples of small populations (59 households) will not yield a sample size sufficient for valid inference. The two groups in the sample were, however, equivalent in origin if not in size. The findings support the weakness in the conceptual framework and in the sample size.

In a study exemplifying an alternative comparative design, Walsh (1985) examined the differences between runners and nonrunners in terms of specific health beliefs. A sample of 150 runners, drawn at random from the membership of a running club, was compared to 150 students randomly chosen from university enrollment. This study demonstrates an alternative to the basic comparative design in the use of a nonequivalent comparison group. In many instances when the design is not an experimental one, it is very difficult to find an equivalent comparison group. Unless another sport is used instead of running, such as tennis or aerobics, it may be impossible to find a comparison group. Because the use of another sport might have confounded the results, these authors elected to draw a random sample of an available population (college students) for comparison. When a comparison group is created in this manner, a complete description of both groups is essential in order to make assessment of the validity of the design possible.

A total of 140 usable questionnaires were returned (46.7%). In the sample, runners tended to be older, with proportionately more males, more marrieds, and higher household incomes than nonrunners. Of the runners, 53% ran every day and 40% ran more than 50 miles a week.

Responses to the Rokeach Health Value Scale (adapted by Wallston) and the Walsh Health Behaviors Questionnaire were analyzed for the 140 subjects. In addition, runners were asked to complete a third questionnaire describing their involvement in running. The two-sample *t*-test for independent groups was used to analyze the data. Findings revealed that runners placed significantly more value on personal health than did nonrunners. In addition, health behaviors differed significantly between the two groups, with runners performing more health-related behaviors than nonrunners in the areas of nutrition, exercise, medical awareness, and self-care.

This study demonstrates an alternative to the basic comparative design in the use of a nonequivalent comparison group. In this case the author was unable to find a comparison group from within the original group, and therefore had to seek a comparison group from an entirely different source. This situation is not unusual in comparative studies. A comparison group could have been found from within another sporting group, but the use of another sport may have confounded the results. To minimize bias, the author drew random samples from two totally different populations: college students and a running club. The size of the two samples was held constant. To allow for assessment of the validity of the design, complete descriptions of both groups were provided.

Flaskerud (1984) compared perceptions of problematic behavior among six minority groups and mental health professionals. The theoretical framework for this study was based on culture. The three components of culture were identified as technology, social structures, and ideology or belief system. The author used this framework to predict the differing responses of the minority groups and the mental health professionals about behavior that could be considered to represent mental illness.

A structured interview format was used with all respondents. Twelve nurse investigators in different parts of the country sampled and interviewed each of the minority and professional groups.

The sample of 227 (68 mental health professionals and 159 minority group members) was selected by convenience. All were 18 years of age or over. The mental health professionals included psychiatrists, psychologists, psychiatric social workers, and psychiatric nurses. There were six minority groups represented: Appalachian, black, Native American, Chinese, Filipino, and Mexican American.

The structured interview schedule had two parts: biographical data and vignettes concerning a person experiencing problems. For each vignette, the subject was asked the following: (1) What do you think of this person's behavior? (2) Do you think anything should be done about it? (3) If so, what? Validity and reliability of the instrument were reported. Responses were dichotomized into mental illness/no mental illness and into psychiatric treatment/no psychiatric treatment. A combined score was derived for each subject on the 10 vignettes, and correlations between sample characteristics and response were examined. A stepwise multiple regression was done to determine the strongest predictor of response.

The results indicated significant differences between the two main groups of mental health professionals and minorities. In addition, minority group status proved to be the strongest predictor of both a mental illness and a psychiatric treatment response, explaining .69 and .72 of the variation, respectively.

This provides an excellent example of a comparative survey testing variables that cannot be examined through experimentation. The author provides a theoretical explanation of the relationship between the variables, although it is not a strong framework and does not result in the usual predictive hypotheses. The study hypotheses are global in nature and merely predict "a difference" between the two main groups. Literature is reviewed relating to each cultural group, but predictions are not made on the basis of cultural group within the general category of minorities. Nevertheless, this study provides an example of comparison based on cultural group, and it is well-designed.

SUITABLE NURSING PROBLEMS

Any study of nurses or patients in natural settings is amenable to the comparative design when the independent variable cannot be manipulated or when it is too early in the research protocol for an experiment. Studies of nursing interventions in natural settings on homogeneous patient populations or on specific inpatient units are an excellent use of this method. Other functional uses for this design include studies of nurse management outcomes in natural settings, patient chart reviews, and comparisons of patient population characteristics (ethnicity, education, geography) with particular health care outcomes.

Comparative designs are hypothesis-testing approaches developed to build support for theory. Because the researcher does not manipulate the independent variable, the major weakness of the design is that it does not control internal validity. Its major strengths are that it provides external validity and allows generalizations to be made, thus testing theory in the field setting where people live and work.

SUMMARY OF THIS DESIGN

In writing a research proposal for this design, the most important issues are related to the basic assumptions underlying the design: (1) The independent variable is not manipulable at this time, if ever, (2) probability sampling techniques are based upon the independent variable, (3) level of measurement of the dependent variable, and (4) the reliability and validity of the instrument(s). (See Chapter 12, on methodological research.)

To summarize, the essential features of this design are as follows:

(1) theoretical framework and predictive hypotheses

(2) representative (probability) sample

(3) accurate measurement of variables

(4) data analysis appropriate to the level of measurement and sample that answers the question, What are the differences between and among the groups?

Any compromise of these basic assumptions constitutes a limitation of the study.

REFERENCES

Cronbach, L. J. (1970). *Essentials of psychological testing* (3rd ed.). New York: Harper & Row.

Flaskerud, J. H. (1984). A comparison of perceptions of problematic behavior by six minority groups and mental health professionals. *Nursing Research, 33*(4), 190-197.

Keane, A., Ducette, J., & Adler, D. C. (1985). Stress in ICU and non-ICU nurses. *Nursing Research, 34*(4), 231-236.

Laffrey, S. C. (1986). Normal and overweight adults: Perceived weight and health behavior characteristics. *Nursing Research, 34*(3), 173-177.

Lynn, M. (1985). Reliability estimates: Use and disuse. *Nursing Research, 34*(4), 254-256.

Munro, B. H., Visintainer, M. A., & Page, E. B. (1986). *Statistical methods for health care research.* Philadelphia: J. B. Lippincott.

Nunnally, J. D. (1978). *Psychometric theory* (2nd ed.). New York: McGraw-Hill.

U.S. Department of Health and Human Services (U.S. DHHS). (1982). *The health consequences of smoking: A report of the surgeon general.* Rockville, MD: Public Health Service.

Walsh, V. R. (1985). Health beliefs and practices of runners versus nonrunners. *Nursing Research, 34*(6), 353-356.

Wildt, A. R., & Ahtola, O. T. (1978). *Analysis of covariance.* Beverly Hills, CA: Sage.

Additional Examples of Studies Using Comparative Designs

LaMontagne, L. L. (1987). Children's preoperative coping: Replication and extension. *Nursing Research, 36*(3), 163-167.

Mynatt, S. (1985). Empathy in faculty and students in different types of nursing preparation programs. *Western Journal of Nursing Research, 7*(3), 333-348.

Ouellette, M. D., MacVicar, M. G., & Harlan, J. (1986). Relationship between percent body fat and menstrual patterns in athletes and non-athletes. *Nursing Research, 35*(6), 330-333.

Reed, P. G. (1986). Developmental resources and depression in the elderly. *Nursing Research, 35*(6), 368-378.

Taylor, M. S., & Covaleski, M. A. (1985). Predicting nurses' turnover and internal transfer behavior. *Nursing Research, 34*(4), 237-241.

5. Correlational Designs

Marilynn J. Wood
Pamela J. Brink

The state of knowledge in many areas within nursing is at the point where the investigator needs to look for relationships among variables. These variables may have been identified in a number of ways. An exploratory study using a qualitative design may have produced a number of variables from a description of a particular patient population. Friesen (1988), for example, in a qualitative study of spouses of patients on home dialysis, identified four categories of spouses. Within these four categories, the variables that appeared to make the difference for the spouse were issues such as level of involvement, marital adjustment, career commitment, and age of children. Alternatively, variables may have come to light during a review of the literature on a particular topic. For example, in a review of disaster studies, Murphy (1987) reports a number of variables that have been suggested to be related to health status in disaster victims. Descriptive studies have also brought to light a number of variables that seem to be related to a given topic. For example, McCloskey and McCain (1988) identified a number of variables related to nurse performance in a study of newly hired nurses at a large midwestern hospital. Identification of variables and determination of their relevance in the study of particular concepts or populations leads to the need to establish more definitive relationships and patterns of relationships in order to begin to explain what is happening in the situation.

A correlational design is used when investigators have reason to suspect a relationship among variables and can support their suspicions through literature or previous research. These variables are known to exist in the population and a conceptual framework can be devised to provide justification for studying them. This design differs from the comparative survey because the framework does not usually have the substance of a theoretical explanation. It merely proposes, based on previous study of the concepts represented by the variables under study, possible connections among these concepts. The purpose of a correlational study is to describe the relationship among the variables, rather than to test theory, but the results may provide support for a particular theoretical perspective, and there is a wide range of situations for which correlational studies are appropriate. These studies vary greatly in the strength of their theoretical bases. On the one hand, though a conceptual framework may be developed to explain possible associations between variables, sometimes the investigator is not sure which variables are independent and which are dependent and may also be unsure of the direction of the relationship. Even if a variable occurs first in time, the investigator may not know whether it directly influences the other variables, whether it is affected by the other variables, or whether any relationship exists at all. This design, therefore, might be used to explore cases where certain variables have associations with one another but the nature of the associations is unknown. In essence, such studies can be "fishing expeditions," although the researcher can always provide at least a tentative conceptual framework to support the examination of these particular variables in the population under study.

On the other hand, an investigator may have a fairly well-developed theoretical framework, but may want to refine the precise relationships among a number of variables. For instance, Mishel and Braden (1987) attempted to delineate the impact of social support on uncertainty in women with gynecologic cancer utilizing a correlational design to determine the relationship among the variables. A model was proposed to predict psychosocial adjustment in the subjects. This study supported the model and the influence of social support and uncertainty on psychosocial adjustment. It is apparent that this design covers a wide range of theoretical perspectives, from tentative conceptual frameworks to well-developed theories. The commonality among these is that in order to progress further, they all require precise description of the relationships among variables.

Correlational designs make use of quantitative data collection methods and multivariate statistical techniques, and may result in the development of causal models. Techniques such as factor analysis, causal modeling, canonical correlation analysis, path analysis, and residual analysis are designed to answer questions about the strength and direction of the relationships among groups of independent and dependent variables, and to generate support for conceptual explanations of variable relationships (Asher, 1983; Berry, 1984; Ferketich & Verran, 1984; Levine, 1977; Thompson, 1984). Because of easy access to computer programs that aid data analysis, these techniques are readily available to researchers. The results are expected to support the development of theory to explain how concepts relate to one another. Correlational designs are at least one step beyond descriptive designs in that the investigator does not examine variables at random, but rather looks at specific variables selected because of the conceptual framework.

There is no control over the independent variables in these designs. All variables are measured as they exist, with no manipulation. In this respect, the correlational design resembles the comparative survey. In the correlational survey, however, the investigator may scrutinize the relationship among several variables without knowing which variables are dependent until data analysis is complete and the results are known.

Complex questions—such as What are the relationships among body weight, body mass index, location of surgery, number and type of previous surgeries, types of anesthesia, gender, intensity and duration of pain, and type, route, and amount of medication among general surgery adult patients?—are appropriately tested using a correlational design. Although body weight, gender, and body mass index all occur first in time, there is no way to predict whether these variables relate in any way to pain perception or medication usage. Although there may be some literature to support the relationship between pain perception and effect of pain medication, there is no theoretical explanation for such a relationship. In addition, the other variables must be assessed to determine whether they enter into the equation. This is a fairly typical question leading to a multiple-variable correlational design.

As pointed out in Chapter 4, early research into the causes of lung cancer used correlational designs to look at broad questions, such as What are the relationships among onset of lung cancer, family history of lung cancer, environmental pollution, diet, smoking, and other personal health habits of U.S. citizens? The dependent variable was known to be lung cancer, so the search was for the independent, intervening, and extraneous variables. The correlational design was chosen to explore the relationships among these variables.

In some correlational research, the independent variable is thought to be known but evidence supporting exactly how it influences other variables is not available. For example, obesity is thought to create a number of different health problems, yet exactly what obesity causes is not really known. In some cases, obesity may actually be a result rather than a cause. Actuarial tables upon which standards for weight by height have been established for the American population have been derived from individuals who carry life insurance. Yet height/weight standards alone without body mass indices, muscle-to-fact ratios, ethnicity, amount or degree of obesity, age of onset of obesity, length of time the subject was obese, placement of adiposity, and age of subject may not be predictive of specific health problems. A correlational design would therefore be useful for finding other variables, in association with the independent variable, that might account for the variance found in subjects with obesity.

BASIC ASSUMPTIONS UNDERLYING CORRELATIONAL DESIGNS

The following assumptions are implicit in the use of correlational designs:

(1) The study variables have not been shown to covary in previous studies of similar populations.
(2) A conceptual framework can be proposed to support the possibility of relationships among the variables.
(3) There is no tested theory upon which to predict the possible relationships among the variables.
(4) The variables exist in the population and are amenable to study.
(5) The sample is representative of the population.
(6) Each variable can be measured accurately with a numerical scale.
(7) There is no manipulation of variables; they are studied as they exist naturally.

BASIC OR CLASSICAL DESIGN

The classic correlational design includes all of the following: a large random sample of the population is assembled; a conceptual framework is proposed to explain potential relationships; research questions, rather than hypotheses, are posed regarding possible relationships among the variables; cross-sectional data are collected on each variable from each subject; data are measured using tools designed to measure quantitative or numerical data; and correlational analysis is used to examine the relationships among the variables. It may be necessary to develop tools to measure some of the variables if no tools are available. In this case, a methodological study is combined with, or done prior to, the correlational survey in order to provide accurate measurement of the variables.

The best sample for a correlational study is a large random sample of the population. The same is a critical element in all designs, but in a correlational design it is of utmost importance that the sample be representative. The whole idea of a correlational study is to determine whether changes in one variable correspond to changes in another variable. The relationships that emerge have no meaning if they cannot be generalized from the sample to a population. The representativeness of the sample, therefore, determines the value of a correlational design, and a large random sample is the best means of ensuring representativeness.

Another issue in the basic correlational design is the conceptual framework. It has already been noted that the investigator does not usually have a theoretical foundation to explain the relationships among the variables under study. However, it is important to develop a possible explanation for covariation among the variables to support the need for the study. It helps to place the study in perspective among other nursing studies, and to justify asking the subjects to participate. It is possible, for example, to consider seeking a correlation between the intellectual performance of elementary school children and the prenatal nutrition of their mothers. But unless a fairly strong case can be built for a direct relationship between these two variables that would still exist in school-aged children in spite of all the intervening events since the prenatal state, it would not be worthwhile to ask mothers and children to invest time and energy providing data for the study. The relationship postulated in this example could be biological, or it could be psychosocial in nature. If no conceptual framework is provided, there is no indication of where this study might fit in the universe of nursing research, and thus the value of the study is questionable. Unless a conceptual framework can be developed, an exploratory descriptive study could handle this topic much more effectively by exploring *all* family variables in a group of elementary school children.

Since the conceptual framework for the correlational survey is usually one posed by the investigator and not one that has been tested in other studies, it makes better sense to summarize the framework in the form of questions rather than hypotheses for study. This supports the tentative nature of the framework and does not give it the appearance of unwarranted strength. The research questions can easily be converted to null hypotheses for statistical testing, without giving them the stature of predictive hypotheses. Predictive hypotheses, then, can be left for designs that actually test theory. Occasionally, a correlational design will be used to test theory when the investigator wishes to look at the interactions among multiple variables as part of theory development. In these cases, the design will be supported by a theoretical framework, and the study integrated into a series of studies planned for testing a particular theoretical perspective.

The data for this design must be primarily quantitative because of the necessity of statistically testing for significant relationships. In the basic design, the data are collected cross-sectionally. At one data collection period, the investigator measures all variables on all subjects and then tests them statistically, looking for significant relationships. No attempt is made to manipulate any of the variables, but all are measured as they exist. One of the strengths of this design is its ability to look at the interaction among several variables at the same time and to see which of them vary together.

Common Variations in the Classical Design

In studies where the researcher is unable to use a random sample, systematic sampling techniques or convenience samples may be used. Remember, this design will be judged on the representativeness of the sample. When nonprobability sampling is used, the researcher must provide detailed information about the sample to allow others to assess its representativeness. External validity in this case would come under question.

Time-series designs can be developed to look at changes in the variables over time. These can be done retrospectively or prospectively, and are sometimes used to predict future events. Using this technique, variables such as changes in health care beliefs can be studied over generations. Ostrom (1978) has provided an in-depth discussion of regression analysis as it applies to time-series designs. This classic work is an excellent guide for designing a correlational study using a time-series approach, because the quality of the inferences drawn from the results will depend heavily on the researcher's having met the assumptions of the time-series analysis.

CONTROL OVER THE DATA

Woods (1985) studied the relationship of socialization and stress to perimenstrual symptoms, disability, and menstrual attitudes. The researcher looked at perimenstrual symptoms (PS) as symptoms rather than disease, from the standpoint of illness behavior and understanding how people adapt to recurring, cyclic symptoms. The purpose of the study was to assess the extent to which a woman's environment and socialization influence her experiences of PS, related disability, and menstrual attitudes.

The study population resided in five neighborhoods in a southeastern U.S. city and consisted of women who were 18 to 35 years old, who were not pregnant, and who had not had hysterectomies. Of 241 potential subjects, 179 agreed to participate. The instruments used to measure the variables were as follows:

(1) Moos Menstrual Distress Questionnaire (MDQ)
(2) 42-item Schedule of Recent Events (SRE)
(3) 16-item Index of Sex Role Orientation (ISRO)
(4) debilitation scale from the Menstrual Attitudes Questionnaire (MAQ)

Path analysis used a multiple regression procedure to test the relationships among stressful life events (STR), socialization (SOC), menstrual attitudes (DE), and disability (DI) for three groups of symptoms: negative affect (NA), pain (PN), and water retention (WR). Pain was first regressed on STR and SOC, then NA on STR and SOC, and WR on STR and SOC. Finally, DI on STR, SOC, PN, NA, and WR and DE on STR, SOC, PN, NA, WR, and DI were regressed. All predictor variables were entered into the equations simultaneously.

Simple correlations for all variables were reported. Stressful life events were positively related to negative affect, and nontraditional socialization was negatively related to debilitation scores. Women who scored high on one symptom scale tended to score high on others. Perimenstrual pain and NA were positively related to DI and DE scores; WR was unrelated to either.

A path model was developed among the concepts that indicated that socialization plays a minor role in explaining severity of perimenstrual symptoms, but traditional socialization was shown to be related to seeing menstruation as debilitating. The influence of a stressful social milieu was important for negative affect symptoms but had only a minor influence on water retention and pain symptoms. Of all symptom clusters, negative affect was most influential with respect to disability.

This report provides an excellent example of a correlational survey that results in the proposal of a causal model. The major assumptions of a correlational design are met. There is a well-developed conceptual framework, which is proposed as a theoretical model because of the relationships found in the study. The sample was randomly selected and should provide accurate representation of the population. Several variables were measured on each subject, and these are examined first to establish their correlations with each other, and then a path analysis mdoel is used to examine the pattern of their relationships to each other as independent and dependent variables and to determine whether or not this pattern supports the conceptual framework. The author explains that a longitudinal study is currently under way to determine whether these causal models will be confirmed. The conceptual framework for this study was chosen from a large number of possibilities representing the immense variability in the research in the area of perimenstrual symptoms and the multitude of theoretical explanations from different fields of study.

In a different study, Majewski (1986) examined the relationship between the maternal role for woman and other roles they may occupy concurrently. This study was based on a conceptual framework derived from role and family development theories, in particular, the idea that role conflict may create a problem for women who occupy several roles—such as spouse and mother roles in addition to occupational roles. This concept was explored in relation to the developmental stage of expansion in which children are born and raised.

The sample consisted of 86 first-time mothers between 20 and 39 years old, currently married, living with spouse, and with a live firstborn infant between 5 and 18 months of age. The sample was nonrandom, consisting of recruits from a variety of agencies and institutions.

Data from a semistructured interview were used to measure transition to the maternal role on a 7-item scale adapted from Blank and Mercer (TMRS). Role conflict was measured using a scale developed by Holahan and Gilbert (RCS). Marital satisfaction was measured with a scale adapted from Roach (MSS). The Employment Role Attitude Scale (ERAS) was developed by Parry and Warr for use with mothers of young children.

The results revealed no significant differences between employed and unemployed mothers on role conflict. This did not differ when work was divided into "career" versus "job." There was, however, a significant relationship for all mothers between perceived role conflict and ease of transition into the maternal role. This correlation was significant for all subscales of the RCS (spouse versus parent, spouse versus self, parent versus self). In addition, there was a significant correlation between perceived marital satisfaction and ease of transition into the maternal role for all mothers. No relationship was found between employment role attitude and ease of transition into the maternal role.

This report provides a good example of a correlational survey that does not use a random sample and in which the independent and dependent variables are not clearly distinguishable. In the analysis of data, transition into the maternal role is presumed to be the dependent variable, yet there is no theoretical foundation for this assumption, as this variable could as easily be the independent variable affecting marital satisfaction, role conflict, and employment satisfaction. Role conflict is used by Majewski as both an independent and a dependent variable (independent in relation to transition to the maternal role, and dependent in relation to employment and career versus job orientation). Thus the "fishing expedition" orientation of the correlational survey is nicely illustrated by this study.

Suitable Nursing Problems

An enormous number of studies can be done using this design. Any study that looks at the interaction between the patient and the institutional environment can be done with a correlational design. For example, studies about the institutional care of Alzheimer patients that look at such elements as level and intensity of noise, colors, and number of people in the environment in relation to selected patient behaviors have yielded new nursing care plans for this group entirely different from the care and environment of other geriatric problems. Specific nursing diagnoses would benefit from correlational studies of the antecedent conditions. Studies examining variables such as social support, locus of control, spiritual well-being, ethnic background, and coping mechanisms of both patients and nurses are appropriate for the correlational design. In nursing education, studies of student characteristics and progress through educational programs are suitable correlational studies. Studies of staffing patterns, nursing care delivery systems, and job satisfaction, burnout, and turnover are good examples of administrative studies using correlational designs. We have just begun to touch on the wealth of questions that need to be addressed using this design. Much of our body of knowledge in nursing is at the level where this is the design of choice.

Studies using correlational designs are classified as descriptive studies because they do not manipulate any variables and do not primarily test theory, but study and describe variables as they exist naturally. These types of studies frequently are based upon findings from single-variable studies. The results contribute to the development of theory.

Samples

The size of the sample is directly related to the number of variables being studied. The sample must be large enough to make possible the documentation of the full range of variance on all the variables, and must fit the assumptions of the data analysis technique that will be used. The need for a representative sample in order to maximize external validity has been noted. The sample selection is a critical element in a correlational survey. The population itself must first be determined to contain all the relevant variables, then the sample size calculated to provide adequate numbers for measurement of the variables; the researcher must bear in mind that a large sample will be more representative than a small one.

Methods of Data Collection

Measurement must be numeric, preferably at the interval or ratio level, although ordinal and nominal data are frequently used. The methods of data collection and the procedures used need to be maintained or standardized. The researcher should use tools that have been tested for reliability and validity on similar populations, and should take steps to control anything that may affect reliability of data during data collection. The value of a correlational survey is directly related to the accurate measurement of the variables.

Data Analysis

This is the design for which multivariate statistical techniques were intended. We will discuss a few of the most commonly used techniques. All of these require interval data. When ordinal scales are used to measure variables, they must be at least metric in nature if any of these methods of analysis are to be used. If categorical or dichotomous (nominal) variables are used, the type of statistical analysis that can be used is significantly changed.

Correlational analysis. The correlation coefficient measures the degree of linear association between two variables. This means that increases in one variable will create like increases (or decreases) in the other variable. The correlation coefficient always lies between the values of $+1$ and -1. When the two variables are unrelated, or have little effect on each other, the correlation coefficient will be close to zero. A positive correlation, meaning that increases in one variable are associated with increases in the other variable, will lie somewhere between zero and $+1$. The close to $+1$ the coefficient approaches, the more clearly it can be associated with increases in the other variable. Negative correlation occurs when an increase in one variable is associated with a decrease in another. The correlation coefficient, in this case, would lie somewhere between zero and -1. The correlation coefficient measures only the degree of association between two variables, and does not indicate a cause-and-effect relationship. Though the two variables may appear to affect each other, it is always possible that both could be related to a third variable that has not been considered.

Multiple correlation. Correlation, as described in the previous paragraphs, is used to test the degree of linear association between two variables: one independent (X) and one dependent (Y). Multiple correlation extends this concept to include relationships between more than one independent variable ($X1$, $X2$, and so on) and one dependent variable (Y). In multiple correlation, the coefficient can range from zero to +1. There are no negative correlations because the method of least squares is used to calculate the correlation coefficient. Multiple correlation is used to measure the relationship between a dependent variable and a weighted combination of independent variables (Munro, Visintainer, & Page, 1986, p. 82).

Regression analysis. Linear regression analysis is used to test the validity of functional relationships. A functional relationship exists where one variable is thought to be affected by changes in another. Regression uses the correlation between variables to make predictions about one variable based on what is known about another. For example, the statement, "The stress level of hospitalized patients is greater when they are unsure of their diagnoses" reflects an inference that stress level is a function of uncertainty in hospitalized patients. Regression analysis assumes that the relationship between stress and uncertainty is linear—that is, an increase in uncertainty creates a proportional increase in stress, so that if the scores were depicted on a graph they would show a straight line with an upward slope. Correlational analysis tells us the amount of variance the two variables share. In regression analysis, however, we can determine whether the actual scores we obtain from our sample on the two variables, uncertainty and stress, are sufficiently close to forming a straight line to support the idea of a functional relationship between them. Linear regression requires that one variable be specifically designated as the dependent variable, and that the variables be measured on interval scales. Ordinal variables can be used if they are continuous (not categorical).

Multiple regression. Linear regression, as discussed above, deals with one independent and one dependent variable. If the study is based on a conceptual framework proposing that several factors might simultaneously affect a dependent variable, multiple linear regression analysis provides a means of measuring the effects of several factors concurrently. According to Schroeder et al. (1986), "The concept is the same as that of simple linear regression except that two or more independent variables are used simultaneously to explain variations in the dependent variable" (p. 30). The results will indicate the effect of any given independent variable on the dependent variable while holding the effects of the other independent variables constant. It is a method of recognizing that multiple factors may influence an observed process, and measuring the relative effect of each factor.

Factor analysis. Factor analysis actually includes statistical techniques, the goal of which is to determine if a large number of variables can be represented by a smaller number of underlying concepts or factors. In a correlational study, the investigator may have measured a number of variables thought to be predisposing to obesity on each member of the sample. It is not known whether there are underlying dimensions to the data that would reduce the number of variables into some common factors, but factor analysis will determine whether there are such underlying dimensions to the data. If they exist, these factors, rather than the individual variables, are assumed to be the actual causes of obesity. Factor analysis provides a way of examining the data to ascertain the minimum number of hypothetical factors that can account for the covariation among the variables (Kim & Mueller, 1978). This use of factor analysis is exploratory, and may result in the development of a theoretical explanation for the covariance among the variables.

Factor analysis can also be used to test a more fully developed conceptual framework. The investigator can hypothesize that there are three underlying dimensions to the data, and that specific variables belong to each of these three dimensions. In this case, factor analysis is used to test theory, rather than to develop it, and the results will show the degree to which the predicted underlying factors actually account for the observed covariation among the variables.

Reliability and Validity

In correlational designs, the concepts of reliability and validity take on critical importance. Since the outcome of the study is determined by the statistical analysis of the data, the measurement of each variable must produce an accurate representation of the true value of the trait being measured. Instrument development, as described by Mishel in Chapter 12, is an important prerequisite of all studies at this level. In addition to using instruments with documented validity and reliability, reliability estimates should be established for all instruments with the population under study. This can be done in a pilot study, or these estimates can be calculated using the study data.

Human Subjects

If the major method of data collection is through the use of questionnaires, personal issues may be raised, leading to self-discovery that may be unpleasant for the subjects. This possibility must always be considered when studying variables representing personal attributes. The investigator should be prepared to assist subject with feelings about self-revelation. In a study that can be viewed as a fishing expedition, there should be a sufficiently sound conceptual framework to warrant asking subjects to contribute their time and energy to providing data for the research. Along these same lines, the design should be sound, as it is an infringement on the rights of subjects to waste their time contributing to a study that is based on a flawed design. Studies that have correlational designs frequently use questionnaires, and are therefore thought to be exempt from review by institutional review boards. This is a practice that should be considered carefully by colleges and universities because of the exploratory nature of some correlational studies. Research subjects have a right to expect that their time and effort is not being wasted by inferior designs that are unlikely to produce any usable results.

RESEARCH PROPOSAL

An adequate conceptual framework is necessary for a correlational survey. Attention must be paid to the establishment of reliability and validity for the instruments. An adequate description of the population and the sampling procedures to be used will provide evidence of a representative sample, ensuring external validity. An adequate description of each tool to be used should be included, along with a rationale for its use, and a relationship should be established between each tool and the study's conceptual framework. The data analysis techniques must be appropriate for establishing relationships among the variables and should be chosen carefully in light of the kind of data (level of measurement) and sample available (sample selection techniques) for the study.

CRITIQUE

A critique of a correlational survey should focus on two areas: sample and measurement. A large random sample of the population forms the basis for this design, and any deviation from this ideal will serve to limit the study. In the area of measurement, those conducting a critique will look for precise quantitative measurement and for the use of instruments that have demonstrated reliability and validity for the population under study.

Essential Features of This Design

In summary, the essential features of a correlational design are as follows:

(1) a large random sample of the population
(2) accurate (valid and reliable) date
(3) multiple measurements on each subject
(4) statistical analysis appropriate to interpretation of the findings

REFERENCES

Asher, H. B. (1983). *Causal modeling* (2nd ed.). Beverly Hills, CA: Sage.
Berry, W. D. (1984). *Nonrecursive causal models*. Beverly Hills, CA: Sage.
Ferketich, S. L., & Verran, J. A. (1984). Residual analysis for causal model assumptions. *Western Journal of Nursing Research, 6*(1), 41-60.
Friesen, D. (1988). *Experience of spouses of dialysis patients*. Unpublished master's thesis, University of Alberta.
Kim, J.-O., & Mueller, C. W. (1978). *Introduction to factor analysis: What it is and how to do it*. Beverly Hills, CA: Sage.
Levine, M. S. (1977). *Canonical analysis and factor comparison*. Beverly Hills, CA: Sage.
Majewski, J. L. (1986). Conflicts, satisfactions, and attitudes during transition to the maternal role. *Nursing Research, 35*(1), 10-14.
McCloskey, J. C., & McCain, B. (1988). Variables related to nurse performance. *Image, 20*(4), 203-207.
Mishel, M. H., & Braden, C. J. (1987). Uncertainty: A mediator between support and adjustment. *Western Journal of Nursing Research, 9*(1), 43-57.
Munro, B. H., Visintainer, M. A., & Page, E. B. (1986). *Statistical methods for health care research*. Philadelphia: J. B. Lippincott.
Murphy, S. A. (1987). Self-efficacy and social support. *Western Journal of Nursing Research, 9*(1), 58-73.
Ostrom, C. W., Jr. (1978). *Time series analysis: Regression techniques*. Beverly Hills, CA: Sage.
Schroeder, L. D., Sjoquist, D. L., & Stephan, P. E. (1986). *Understanding regression analysis*. Beverly Hills, CA: Sage.
Thompson, B. (1984). *Canonical correlation analysis*. Beverly Hills, CA: Sage.
Woods, N. F. (1985). Relationship of socialization and stress to perimenstrual symptoms, disability, and menstrual attitudes. *Nursing Research, 34*(3), 145-149.

PART **IV**

EXPLORATORY-DESCRIPTIVE DESIGNS

Exploratory descriptive designs, usually field studies in natural settings, provide the least control over variables. The data collected either contribute to the development of theory or explain phenomena from the perspective of the persons being studied.

There are two major types of *descriptive studies*: those that provide (1) descriptions of a single broad variable in a single population, or (2) descriptions of population characteristics. These studies answer the question, What are the X customs of Y population? or What are the characteristics of X population? These questions result in description of either the population characteristics or the variable. Lack of current knowledge about either the variable or the population precludes the use of a theoretical base for the study, as specific predictions of cause-and-effect relationships cannot be made.

Studies of a single variable previously investigated in one population but not in another are appropriately descriptive. Just because a variable has been studied and described in one population does not necessarily mean that it even exists in another population. Therefore, the first task of a researcher is to find the variable itself, then describe how the variable exists or acts in the new population. Previously studied variables usually form the basis for a theoretical explanation of their action. In this case, descriptive studies of single (previously studied) variables in unknown or understudied populations are usually based upon theory derived from previous research.

A population survey, like the study of a single variable, is atheoretical, and no cause-and-effect relationship is sought and no predictions can be made other than the fact that population characteristics will exist. Such a statement is in fact a basic assumption of the study and therefore not a prediction or the basis of a hypothesis. Two reasons for doing population surveys might be that a similar study may have been done but a fresh perspective is being sought, that an update of an older study is needed to determine if there has been any change over time. In both cases, the studies are cross-sectional descriptions of a population.

Descriptive studies of populations take two perspectives. Population studies reflect the perspective of the investigator, using questionnaires and interviews as the primary data collection methods. In contrast, ethnographies, using multiple data collection methods (participant observation, census, available data, interviews, genealogies, life histories, and demographies) attempt to discover population characteristics from the perspective of the person being studied. Ethology, the minute observation and description of nonverbal behaviors of humans and animals, is purely descriptive. Ethnomethodology, through direct observation and film analysis, attempts to discover the cultural rules underlying everyday behavior and addresses the question, What are the informal rules underlying X behavior or X social interaction? Although descriptive studies attempt to discover the world of the research subject and describe it accurately, the analysis is usually from the perspective of the observer or researcher. Because the analysis is guided by the researcher, the study may be analyzed from the perspective of known theory as well as being purely descriptive in form.

Exploratory studies, on the other hand, have three functions: (1) in-depth exploration and description of a single variable, process, or phenomenon, in order to arrive at complete description and explication; (2) as a feasibility study (also known as a pilot project) to determine whether or not a study plan is feasible as designed (the pilot project will be dealt with separately in another chapter); and (3) as the first phase of a planned long-term research project. In this section we describe only the first and third functions of the exploratory design.

Exploratory designs are commonly employed in an attempt to see the world as the participant or research subject sees it. These designs are often equated with qualitative designs, as they rely on qualitative data collection methods exclusively. Phenomenology, ethnoscience, and grounded theory are the major designs within qualitative research. Grounded theory always assumes process, and aims for a theoretical explanation of how the process works. Ethnoscience uses linguistic analysis to define a situation or abstract concept. Phenomenology seeks to describe the experience of the phenomenon under study (e.g., What does it feel like to be a patient in a hospital?), although the goal is not to discover process as a grounded theory; experience involves process, therefore how one experiences a phenomenon constitutes a description of a process. Ethnoscience, more frequently called "ethnography" by some nurse-anthropologists (Aamodt, 1982), has rigid rules for data analysis based upon repeated observation of natural behaviors, whereas phenomenology and grounded theory are more flexible and more dependent upon the creativity of the researcher in the analysis of data. They are also most likely to use nontraditional sources of data.[1]

The issue of control in exploratory designs is moot, as the situation not the investigator, controls the data. Rather, it is the flexibility of the investigator that is essential in these designs. The investigator must be able to "go with the flow," to abandon an area that is not fruitful or to go in depth into an area not previously planned. Descriptive studies, with their more structured data collection (instrumentation is available in many cases) and more specific samples, afford greater control over measurement than do exploratory studies. The least controlled, most flexible, and most creative study is the exploratory design. Critical to both studies are the step-by-step explication of the sample selection process, the data collection procedures used, and the techniques for data analysis. Because these designs often describe totally uncharted areas, validity and reliability depend on the meticulous use of detailed field notes, selection of field informants, and repeated observations and interviews of the same subject over time.

NOTE

1. We are indebted to Field and Morse (1985) for the clarity of their definitions and descriptions of qualitative research approaches in their text, and we are delighted that they frequently used the question approach to clarify the differences in these designs.

REFERENCES

Aamodt, A. M. (1982). Examining ethnography for nursing researchers. *Western Journal of Nursing Research, 4*(2), 209-222.

Field, P., & Morse, J. (1985). *Nursing research: The application of qualitative approaches.* London: Croom Helm.

6. Descriptive Designs

Pamela J. Brink
Marilynn J. Wood

Part of the development of a complete data base for any science is the detailed description and classification of the various phenomena related to that science. Prior to the manipulation/disruption of any natural phenomena, the researcher spends years in the intimate study of a particular problem. The difficulty for any new science has been the establishment of the phenomena unique to that discipline. The fields of anatomy and physiology began with a painstaking description of gross anatomy based upon detailed and repetitive observations of cadavers. Today, anatomy remains an essentially descriptive science, albeit at the microscopic level. Criminology is based upon the intense study of criminals and their characteristics, and upon detailed study of the interactions between criminals and their victims. The sciences of astronomy, zoology, and botany are also based upon painstaking description and classification. Nursing science similarly requires that any phenomenon first be explored at the qualitative level, then validated through the descriptive design. Thorough exploration and description of a phenomenon must precede the search for relationships between it and other phenomena.

Research studies using the descriptive design include anthropological ethnograpies (descriptions of the social systems of single small societies or culture groups), census studies, and sociological demographies (demographic characteristics of particular populations). A number of descriptive studies in both the natural and social sciences have been featured on television. The work of Jane Goodall, Jacques Cousteau, and of the Leakey family (Louis, Mary, and Richard), and the story

of Lucy are all descriptive field studies. A number of eduational television series, including *The Disappearing World, Nova,* and *River Journeys,*
provide ethnographic (descriptive) accounts of unfamiliar peoples and
places. Descriptive designs are usually, but not always, cross-sectional
and make use of both qualitative and quantitative data collection
methods. The type of method chosen depends upon the sample size
and level of knowledge about the variable and the population. Descriptive research can be either inductive or deductive. For the most part,
however, these terms are not useful, since valid description contributes
to theory building as well as to theory testing.

BASIC OR CLASSICAL DESIGN

There are two major types of descriptive designs. The first is a survey
of population characteristics or a demography of a total available
population. When various characteristics of a particular population are
either unknown or partially (incompletely) known, the design of choice
is the descriptive design. Thus the question, What are the characteristics
of successful dieters? can be answered through a descriptive study.
(Although some may respond, "Easy—they lose weight!" this response
is, in reality, a definition of a successful dieter, not a description of
their common characteristics—not the plural.) Even when there has
been previous research about a variable, a descriptive design may be
used if the researcher wishes to study that varible in a different population. Descriptions of the characteristics of men may or may not apply
to women. But until the characteristics of women are also described
for the same variables, knowledge of both sexes is limited. The critical
point is that the variable in question either has not been studied (or
reported) previously for a particular population or was reported long
enough ago to warrant a new study.

The second type of descriptive design involves the complete description of a single broad variable or concept within a given population.
Again, the variable should be either unstudied or understudied in that
population. Examples of descriptive questions on single variables include: What are the health beliefs of the Amish of Iowa? What are the
value orientations of the Annang of Nigeria? (Brink, 1984), and What
types of birth defects occur among infants of teenage mothers? Complete description of specific phenomena within a population is critical

to theory building (inductive) as well as to theory testing (deductive). Descriptive studies contribute to both purposes. For example, the work of Florence Kluckhohn served the purpose of contributing to anthropological knowledge about human nature, and was inductive in its beginning stages. Florence Kluckhohn lived on or near a Navajo reservation for many summers, using participant observation. From her observations she began to develop a concept of human nature as a series of societal decisions in relation to values. Kluckhohn felt that all human groups need to solve certain common human problems, and that the way a society solves its problems reflects what it values and believes. These values and beliefs are amenable to discovery through questioning. Based upon her theory, Kluckhohn and Strodtbeck (1961) developed and tested the Value Orientation instrument on five cultural groups in the southwestern United States. The configuration of value orientations obtained by means of Kluckhohn's instrument constituted a description of a particular cultural group. Because Kluckhohn developed an instrument to test her theory, the resulting descriptive research was deductive. Using the same instrument, Brink (1984) described the value orientations of the Annang of Nigeria, thus extending the knowledge of the same variable in a different population. The Brink study, although a purely deductive descriptive study, contributes to the original Kluckhohn theory.

A purely descriptive study reported by McIver at the 1985 Council of Nurse Researchers meetings in San Diego was based upon the question: "What are the symptoms reported by menopausal women?" She interviewed over 100 women, many of them several times, to discuss their experiences during and post-menopause and to discover their common symptomatology. Once the data had been analyzed and categories derived, McIver was able to report symptomatology (e.g., breast pain) very common among this population that had never been reported in the literature. She was not interested in building a theory about menopause; rather, she was concerned with a more complete description of this population.

BASIC ASSUMPTIONS UNDERLYING DESCRIPTIVE DESIGNS

The following assumptions are implicit in the use of descriptive designs:

(1) The variable exists in the population under study, and it is a single variable amenable to description.

(2) There is little or no literature that describes the current population (or variable) at the present time.

(3) There may be no theoretical framework for the study, but a detailed rationale for the research based upon a thorough literature review is necessary.

(4) There may be a theoretical or conceptual framework underlying the study, as in the case of a known concept being studied in a new population. Previous research provides the rationale and framework for the present study.

(5) When the population parameters are unknown, and the basic criteria for external validity cannot be met through sample selection procedures, the findings cannot be generalized from the sample to the population.

(6) When population parameters are known, and the basic criteria for external validity can be met through sample selection procedures, population parameters can be estimated from sample measures.

A number of classic descriptive designs have emerged from different disciplines. These classic designs include demography, ethnography, ethnomethodology, content analysis, population census, opinion polls, ethology, ethnographic semantics or ethnoscience, descriptive linguistics, and archaeology. Each of these designs can be distinguished according to (1) whether a population (ethnography, demography, census) or a variable (ethnomethodology, ethnoscience, content analysis) is to be described, and (2) whether the data collection method is observation (ethology, archaeology), questioning (ethnomethodology, ethnoscience, descriptive linguistics), available data (content analysis, archaeology), or a combination of many methods (ethnography). All these designs appear to fit at least one of our two basic attributes of descriptive designs: a description of a single broad variable within a specific population (ethnoscience, ethology, archaeology) or a description of the characteristics of a population as a whole (ethnography, census, demography).

CONCEPTUAL FRAMEWORK

Descriptive studies frequently lack a conceptual framework; the rationale for the study therefore becomes critical. The investigator must explain, for example, how the research might promote the development of nursing knowledge and how the results might lead to further work. Without such rationales, descriptive studies tend to appear insignificant, are unlikely to be funded by granting agencies, and are unlikely to be published once completed. Only in this area does a descriptive design proposal differ from proposals using other designs.

CONTROL OVER DATA

Control over data is limited in descriptive designs. The setting is essentially uncontrolled or outside the control of the investigator. The investigator exerts some control over sample selection when drawing a representative sample from the population. Descriptive studies always examine the variable/sample as it exists, without investigator interference.

SAMPLING

The ideal sample for a descriptive design is either a total available population (particularly with small populations) or a sample drawn by means of probability sampling techniques from a target population. If the purpose of a study is to describe population characteristics, probability sampling techniques are necessary to ensure external validity. The U.S. census employs a descriptive design that uses both systematic sampling techniques (for in-depth data collection of 10% of the population) and total available population (for a comprehensive description of the population characteristics). Frequently, however, population parameters are not available and probability sampling cannot be used, thereby creating problems for external validity. Internal validity is not an issue in descriptive designs because no attempts are made to examine causal relationships among variables.

METHODS OF DATA COLLECTION

Data collection methods include observation, questioning, available data, projective techniques, physical assessment or physiological tests of humans, and chemical or physical tests on nonhumans or inanimate objects. Studies may utilize a single in-depth method such as intensive interviewing, or combinations of structured and semistructured methods (structured interviews coupled with participant observation, collection of written and unwritten available data, oral histories, genograms and kinship charts, cartography, multiple physical specimens or measurements, still and moving photographs, recordings of music). Data in census studies are usually collected through interview and/or questionnaire (Fink & Koseocoff, 1985). Descriptive studies of single variables are usually grounded in ethnographic accounts of a single culture or group. Ethnographies (e.g., Agar, 1980; Ellen, 1984; Field & Morse, 1985; Germain, 1986; Hammersley & Atkinson, 1983; Pelto & Pelto, 1978), also called fieldwork (Wax, 1971; Werner, 1987; Whiting et al., 1966; Whyte, 1984), rely on a combination of data collection methods, usually including all of the following: participant observation (McCall & Simmons, 1969), available data (Pelto & Pelto, 1978; Stewart, 1984), intensive interviewing (Agar, 1986; Spradley, 1979), census, kinship charts (Crane & Angrosino, 1984), life histories, and photographic and audiotape evidence. The data collection instruments used for ethnographies are predominantly structured and semistructured rather than unstructured, reflecting an important difference between descriptive and exploratory designs. In some instances, the variable under study can be found only in data such as hospital charts, newspapers, or data collected for other purposes (including other research studies). These descriptive studies are thus based upon available data, and the task of the researcher is to sort the data into some logical taxonomic form (see Hunter & Foley, 1976; Krippendorf, 1980). Animal field studies yield a great deal of photographic material upon which secondary analysis can be based. Nurses' notes, nursing care plans, and published articles are all grist for the available data descriptive study.

A frequent method of data collection is questioning, in the form of either interviews or questionnaires (Spradley, 1979). The vignette technique used in the Kluckhohn and Strodtbeck (1961), Flaskerud (1980), and Brink (1984) studies to elicit culturally based belief systems is both a highly structured data collection device and a projective test of underlying values and beliefs. Hayter (1983) developed questionnaires based on sleep behaviors documented in younger populations, then modified the questionnaires to allow for differences that might be present in an older group. Archer's (1983) study of political participation, on the other hand, merely collected demographic data on the population using structured tools related to political behavior.

Observational techniques can also be used, particularly participant observation (McCall & Simmons, 1969). Many descriptive studies of natural phenomena rely exclusively on direct but nonparticipant field observations, especially in fields such as archaeology, astronomy, and field primatology. Mixed methods are also used frequently. Since the knowledge base is so uncertain, the researcher may not be sure which method will be best or most efficient for data collection.

The relevance of the data collection method to the population must be considered. For example, interviewing individuals to ask them what they do in particular situations must be validated through the use of observational techniques to see if respondents actually do what they say they do in those situations. If, on the other hand, the sample is being asked about beliefs, personal history, or personal facts, observational techniques would not be useful. In this case, interviews with other knowledgeable people to support or refute subjects' statements can be valuable.

In a descriptive study based entirely upon questionnaire or interview data collection instruments, the questions, and the order in which they are asked, are completely planned before any interviewing takes place. In other words, the degree of flexibility needed in an exploratory study is not appropriate for a descriptive study. For example, in some exploratory studies, the investigator asks questions as they are conceived. The questions, as well as their order, may differ from subject to subject. In descriptive designs, this flexibility is not allowed. This structure gives the researcher control over the data insofar as questions are standardized, and are asked in a standardized order.

The type of question asked can be either semistructured or structured. A semistructured question is one in which the question is standardized and the order in which the question is asked is preset, but answers are open and unstructured. Examples of semistructured questions include the following:

- *Grand tour questions* (Spradley & McCurdy, 1972) (setting the tone for the interview or questionnaire): "I would like you to tell me about the last time you gave birth. Just begin at the beginning, when you began to have labor pains, start from there."
- *Complete the sentence:* "People should abstain from alcohol and drugs because . . ."

- *Fill in:* "I believe nurses _____ every day."
- *Contrast or comparative questions:* "Tell me what you think are the differences between men and women in relation to their ability to be successful weight losers. In what way are they similar? In your opinion, who would have the most difficulty being a successful weight loser?"
- *Inclusive questions:* "What kinds of people become drug addicts?" Or, "If you were on the admissions committee of a school of nursing, what qualities would you insist applicants have?" Or, "What are the qualities or characteristics of a *good* nurse?"
- *Exclusive questions:* "If you were to develop a new community program in eldercare, who would not be eligible?" Or, "What kinds of research would you say are not nursing research?" Or, "What kinds of problems are not health problems?"

The smaller the sample size, the larger the number of unstructured questions that can be included. One of the reasons for this is that unstructured questions usually lead to large amounts of unstructured data that must be put into some sensible format. If one person is asked to tell a life history in one or two hours, the amount of data to be transcribed and analyzed will be enormous. Two people answering the same question with the same amount of data will yield twice the complexity of analysis—three even more so, and so on. Investigators find that large amounts of unstructured data can be unwieldy, and that some mechanism for analysis through the use of computers becomes necessary. Because few computer programs now available on the market can handle this type of data, investigators limit the number of people in the sample rather than the amount of data from each person.

The opposite is equally true: The larger the sample, the more structured the questions need to be, and the fewer the unstructured questions allowable. This results partially from computer-assisted analysis of data, in which numerical answers can be entered easily into a computer and statistically manipulated. The more numerical answers in a questionnaire or observational checklist, the more easily the data can be prepared for computer analysis.

Examples of structured questions on an ordinal scale include the following:

- *Multiple choice:* Which of the following best represents your family income level? Select only one answer.

(a) $ 0-4,999 per year
(b) $ 5,000-9,999 per year
(c) $10,000-19,999 per year
(d) $20,000-29,999 per year
(e) $30,000 or more per year

- *Likert scale:* Check the one response that best describes how you feel about the statement: "Alcoholism is basically a character disorder."

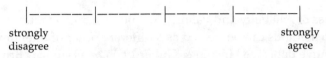

strongly
disagree

strongly
agree

Please rate how well the following statement fits your belief about abortion: "Abortion is an act of murder."

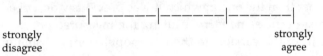

strongly
disagree

strongly
agree

- *Ranking:* Which three of the following life events have been most difficult for you? Please rank your three choices in order, from the most difficult (1) to the least difficult (3).
  - _____ (1) childhood
  - _____ (2) marriage
  - _____ (3) retirement
  - _____ (4) illness of self or spouse
  - _____ (5) death of spouse or other close relative
  - _____ (6) children leaving home
  - _____ (7) parenthood
  - _____ (8) other (please specify)

Some seemingly open-ended fill-in questions are, in reality, highly structured, metric-scale questions. For example, when you ask an individual, "How old are you?" and provide a fill-in blank, the answer will be given in numerical years. Numbers or numerical answers of this kind are considered structured questions, as are fill-in answers requiring blood pressure readings, temperature, and pulse, despite the fact that a fill-in blank is provided. In this case only a number is expected.

Whether questions are structured or semistructured, the purpose is to be as standardized as possible at this stage of the research in order to analyze the answers to each individual question as a unit in and of itself using descriptive statistics. Later analysis (using tests of association or correlation depending upon the type of question) might attempt to show an association between the answers from one question and one or more other questions or the demographic data.

RELIABILITY AND VALIDITY

Issues of reliability and validity in studies using qualitative data collection methods can be treated as a different order of phenomena than qualitative data (see Lincoln & Guba, 1985) or as similar (Brink, 1989). Instruments developed in one population may prove unreliable or invalid in another. For example, the variable may not exist in a population other than the one in which it was previously described; or it may not exist in the same form, causing the measurement to miss critical elements of the variable in the new population. Reliability and validity of the source of the data are also important. Lack of knowledge about the population can lead an investigator to make serious errors in designing the study. This possibility makes pretesting of all tools essential. *Aquiescent response set* (in which certain individuals always tend to agree with the interviewer) and *social desirability* (in which people tend to answer according to what they think is the socially correct answer rather than the actual answer, which may make them look silly or stupid) are validity issues that need to be addressed, particularly when the respondent must choose from a series of alternatives. These traits may be more prominent in an unknown culture than the investigator expects. Depending upon who else is present in an interview session, social desirability can be a confounding factor in any culture. When the investigator is seen as having high social status, or when the interviewer is thought to be connected with the police or other law enforcement, as in the case of interviewing illegal aliens, social desirability becomes especially problematic.

There are two standard methods of ensuring the reliability and validity of data in descriptive studies: (1) the use of repeated interviews over time on the same subject; and (2) the use of observations in conjunction with interviews. In the first instance the researcher tests the stability of the informants' statements. Since it is difficult to tell an untruth over and over again on a variety of topics, repeated interviews with a single informant yield reliable data in the end. While interviewing the informant in a natural setting, the researcher usually asks for interpretations and/or explanations of what is going on in that setting at the time of the interview. The researcher observes the social scene, then asks the informant for an explanation. The researcher can also ask informants what they do in particular situations, and then observe them in those situations to see if, indeed, their reports were accurate. Such validation procedures are a necessary requisite to descriptive designs utilizing either interviewing or observation. When a descriptive design utilizes available data, the researcher can return to the data again and again to make certain that the data base elicited from the written material is correct. Such repeated readings may also yield new insights into the material that were not immediately apparent on the first reading. To validate these new insights, the researcher can ask a second person to review the materials, given this new definition; that person can tell the researcher if the material supports the new conclusions.

DATA ANALYSIS

Methods of analysis will differ according to the type of study, the sampling procedures, and the degree of complexity of data collection methods. The least complex study would involve one type of data collection method—whether questioning, observation, or available data—and one level of measurement in a predominantly structured data collection instrument supplemented with a few semistructured items. A more complex study would involve a combination of data collection methods and a combination of levels of measurement within and across methods, resulting in a mixture of structured and unstructured data, a mixture of nominal, ordinal, and metric-scale data, and a mixture of informational sources.

When data are semistructured or unstructured, data analysis begins with content analysis (Krippendorf, 1980; Miles & Huberman, 1984; Wilson, 1985, Chap. 14), separating the answers to each question into mutually exclusive categories of similar content. The first step in content analysis is to read all answers to each question several times in order to establish a "feel" for the answers. As each answer is read, a "general sense" of the implication of the answers is established, producing a beginning formulation of possible contrasting categories of content. An initial attempt is made to separate all content into these initial categories. During this process, subcategories of content within each of the original categories become apparent, and a second analysis is begun based upon the new categorization of mutually exclusive contrast material. At each step, the decisions or rules guiding separation of content are written down. Eventually all the data will be accounted for in some category. The number of responses within each category and subcategory can be tabulated and frequencies can be reported on that tabulation.

Also basic to this design are descriptive statistics (frequencies, percentages, means, medians, and modes) including standard deviations, quartiles, and ranges. If the collected data already exist in numerical form, the first step in analysis is to summarize the responses to each question. For nominal data, this will include simple frequencies and modes; for ordinal data, it includes frequencies, ranges, and medians; and for interval and ratio data, frequencies, variances, and means. Interval and ratio data can also be described in relation to ranges, standard deviations, and quartiles.

In studies of population characteristics, sample statistics are used to predict population parameters. It is possible, therefore, to estimate the incidence of disease or other health problems in the population from data collected from a random sample.

When the study calls for nonprobability sampling and/or when measurement is at the nominal or ordinal level, nonparametric statistics are used. Whether the study is of a single variable or of a population as a whole, simple tests of association are helpful as an aid to discovering whether or not there are any indicators for further research on the same or other populations. The question to be answered is, Is there any association between the answers to any of the individual questions and any of the population characteristics? When the study is of a single variable, these tests are usually done between the variable under study and the demographic characteristics of the sample. If all data are nominal, or if the major variable is nominal and all other variables are run against a nominal variable, the chi-square test is useful. If ordinal variables are used as the base variable against ordinal or metric data, then Spearman's rho is helpful. Otherwise, the Pearson r is used to test for relationships among metric variables. When the study is of population characteristics as a whole, then all population variables are run against one another (using tests appropriate for the level of measurement) to determine whether there are any associations worth following up in another study.

HUMAN SUBJECTS ISSUES

Human subjects issues vary widely. In ethnographic studies, the subjects' lack of understanding of the research process may present problems. In this case, issues of *informed consent* are very important, as explanation of the research in terms the subject can understand is critical. In participant observation studies, the issues are the same as those in qualitative research. In census studies, the major ethical concerns include confidentiality of the data and anonymity of the subjects.

EXAMPLES OF DESCRIPTIVE DESIGNS

Archer (1983) designed a study to provide baseline data on nursing administrators' participation in policymaking processes. A random sample of 1,086 nurse administrators from community health agencies, home health agencies, hospitals, and schools of nursing was drawn for the study, according to the following proportionate design:

(1) all directors of public health nursing services of state and territorial health departments
(2) five directors of local public health nursing services, randomly selected from each state and territory
(3) five directors of home health agencies, randomly selected from each state's list of member agencies in the NLN Council of Home Health Agencies and Community Health Services
(4) seven directors of hospital nursing services, randomly selected from each state's and territory's list of Joint Commission Accredited Hospitals with more than 200 beds
(5) three deans, randomly selected from NLN-accredited baccalaureate and higher degree programs in each state and territory

The rationale for sampling was to have each type of institution represented in approximate proportion to its representation in the national agency or institutional population. The instrument for data collection was a self-administered, mailed, anonymous questionnaire developed specifically for this study and extensively pretested to develop face and content validity. Overall political participation for the sample of nursing administrators was relatively high, and is described in detail in the report in the form of a typology of activities. Archer explains that the results may have been influenced by the fact that data collection occurred during a successful campaign to overturn the Nurse Training Act veto. The most common reason given for lack of political participation was deficient understanding and skill in the political process.

This report provides a good example of a descriptive study based on a survey of population characteristics. The author uses a proportionate random sample from carefully defined nursing administration groups that can be generalized to this population of administrators. There is no conceptual framework for the study, but the author explains that political participation in issues related to public policy affecting nursing is part of the professional responsibility of the nurse.

Hayter (1983) studied sleep behaviors of older persons. This study exemplifies how a variable (sleep behaviors) that is well documented in different populations can be studied in a population in which it has not been examined before (older persons). Because of lack of norms for the elderly population, older persons' sleep had been evaluated on the basis of sleep norms for younger adults. The purpose of this study was to determine the nature of sleep behaviors in older persons of different ages.

Two instruments were devised for the study, both based on previous literature on sleep behaviors. The first was a questionnaire designed to supply information about typical sleep behaviors, demographic variables, and daily activities that might affect sleep. The second was a modified version of another researcher's sleep chart, on which subjects marked each 30-minute period they were asleep during each 24-hour period for two weeks. Both instruments were pretested with healthy older persons. A pilot study was conducted to test reliability and validity of the instrument on 22 residents without major health problems at a home for the aged.

The investigator drew a random sample of 325 older persons from a pool of over 1,000 who had given their permission to be contacted as potential subjects for research through a gerontology center. The instruments were mailed to the subjects, along with instructions; 212 subjects returned complete responses.

The findings clearly document a pattern of gradually increasing need for both rest and sleep with advancing age, with the need for increased rest occurring earlier than the need for increased sleep. These data show that certain changes are expected in sleep behaviors with increasing age, and that sleep patterns differ markedly from those of younger people. These findings emphasize the need for documentation of known concepts in unknown populations, and support the idea that patterns that are valid in one population may not be so in another.

In a different type of descriptive design, Flaskerud (1980) compared perceptions of problematic behavior in three different populations. Three groups of respondents (Appalachian laypersons, non-Appalachian laypersons, and mental health professionals) were interviewed using eight vignettes that described various problematic behaviors. The vignettes were developed from actual case histories of Appalachians diagnosed as mentally ill and hospitalized with that diagnosis. Each respondent was asked to label the behavior and suggest appropriate methods of management.

A metropolitan neighborhood that served as an entry point for Appalachian migrants was selected as the available population of lay Appalachians. A sample of 75 households was drawn from a list of 250 houses. To ensure an equal number of men and women in the sample, the sex of the subject selected differed in alternate households. Other criteria for sample selection included age and area from which respondents migrated. A total of 50 households were eligible for inclusion in the study. Mental health professionals were selected from all agencies serving the Appalachian migrant or located within the target neighborhood. The total population of professionals making diagnostic judgments in these agencies were asked to participate, and 54 agreed. Lay non-Appalachians were selected from a random sampling of names from a telephone book listing persons living in an area contiguous to the Appalachian neighborhood. The phone book page, column, and line were all randomly selected. To account for individuals who did not have telephones, the household next to the one selected from the book was included. In the case of multiple units, all units were listed and one selected at random. Of the persons selected by this process, 51 agreed to participate.

Content analysis was used to categorize all labels as mental illness (MI) or non-mental illness (NMI), and all treatments as psychiatric treatment (PT) or as nonpsychiatric treatment (NPT). The composition of the resulting categories was then compared both within and across groups using a one-way analysis of variance. No significant differences were found between mental health professionals and the lay group of non-Appalachians, but significant differences were found between these two groups and the lay Appalachians.

This report provides a good example of a descriptive design that examines a known variable (diagnosis of mental illness) in three different populations, looking for similarities and differences among the three. The findings show that the Appalachian population did not see the behavior described in the vignettes as abnormal, indicating a significant cultural gap. This study differs from a comparative design in its lack of theoretical framework and hypotheses, and in the manner in which the concept of diagnosis of mental illness was measured. The study utilizes random sampling from two of the populations and the total population for the third, thus producing generalizable results. However, because the purpose of this study was to describe the population, we can only speculate about reasons for the findings. The study, therefore, leads to the development of hypotheses for further study.

SUMMARY

Essential features of the descriptive design include the following:

(1) Breadth of data—comprehensive data collection from every conceivable source, using every available method from every available knowledgeable subject—should result in a *complete* description of the variable or the population.
(2) Reliability and validity of the measurements is crucial. When instruments are used for the first time with a population, they must be pretested to establish their reliability and validity. If the data collection instruments are completely unstructured, perhaps the choice of design is incorrect and the study belongs in the qualitative arena.
(3) The sample must be either a total population or a representative sample from a larger population.

Suitable Nursing Problems

The descriptive design is useful for documenting various characteristics in populations of interest to nurses in order to gather baseline data on those populations. Variables such as uncertainty, nutritional status, and depression, for example, could be measured on populations of patients with different diagnoses. In the development of nursing science, patient resources can be described and reported in taxonomies.

REFERENCES

Agar, M. H. (1980). *The professional stranger: An informal introduction to ethnography*. New York: Academic Press.

Agar, M. H. (1986). *Speaking of ethnograpy*. Beverly Hills, CA: Sage.

Archer, S. E. (1983). A study of nurse administrators' political participation. *Western Journal of Nursing Research, 5*(1), 65-75.

Brink, P. J. (1984). Value orientations as an assessment tool in cultural diversity. *Nursing Research, 33*(4), 198-203.

Brink, P. J. (1989). Issues in reliability and validity. In J. M. Morse (Ed.), *Qualitative nursing research: A contemporary dialogue* (pp. 139-154). Rockville, MD: Aspen.

Crane, J. G., & Angrosino, M. V. (1985). *Field projects in anthropology: A student handbook*. Prospect Heights, IL: Waveland.

Ellen, R. F. (1984). *Ethnographic research: A guide to general conduct*. London: Academic Press.

Field, P. A., & Morse, J. M. (1985). *Nursing research: The application of qualitative approaches*. London: Croom Helm.

Fink, A., & Kosecoff, J. (1985). *How to conduct surveys: A step-by-step guide*. Beverly Hills, CA: Sage.

Flaskerud, J. H. (1980). Perceptions of problematic behavior by Appalachians, mental health professionals and lay non-Appalachians. *Nursing Research, 29*(3), 140-149.

Germain, C. (1986). Ethnography: The method. In P. L. Munhall & C. J. Oiler (Eds.), *Nursing research: A qualitative perspective* (pp. 147-162). Norwalk, CT: Appleton-Century-Crofts.

Hammersley, M., & Atkinson, P. (1983). *Ethnography: Principles in practice*. New York: Tavistock.

Hayter, J. (1983). Sleep behaviors in older persons. *Nursing Research, 32*(4), 242-246.

Hunter, D. E., & Foley, M. B. (1976). *Doing anthropology: A student centered approach to cultural anthropology*. New York: Harper & Row.

Kluckhohn, F., & Strodtbeck, F. L. (1961). *Variations in value orientations*. Elmsford, NY: Row, Peterson.

Krippendorf, K. (1980). *Content analysis: An introduction to its methodology*. Beverly Hills, CA: Sage.

Lincoln, Y. S., & Guba, E. G. (1985). *Naturalistic inquiry*. Beverly Hills, CA: Sage.

McCall, G. J., & Simmons, J. L. (Eds.). (1969). *Issues in participant observation: A text and reader*. Reading, MA: Addison-Wesley.

Miles, M. B., & Huberman, A. M. (1984). *Qualitative data analysis: A sourcebook of new methods*. Beverly Hills, CA: Sage.

Pelto, P. J., & Pelto, G. H. (1978). *Anthropological research: The structure of inquiry* (2nd ed.). Cambridge: Cambridge University Press.

Spradley, J. P. (1979). *The ethnographic interview*. New York: Holt, Rinehart & Winston.

Spradley, J. P. (1980). *Participant observation*. New York: Holt, Rinehart & Winston.

Spradley, J. P., & McCurdy, D. W. (1972). *The cultural experience: Ethnography in complex society*. Chicago: Science Research Associates.

Stewart, D. W. (1984). *Secondary research: Information sources and methods*. Beverly Hills, CA: Sage.

Wax, R. (1971). *Doing fieldwork: Warnings and advice*. Chicago: University of Chicago Press.

Werner, O., & Schoepfle, G. M. (1987). *Systematic fieldwork* (2 vols.). Newbury Park, CA: Sage.

Whiting, J. W. M., et al. (1966). *Field guide for a study of socialization*. New York: John Wiley.
Whyte, W. F. (1984). *Learning from the field: A guide from experience*. Beverly Hills, CA: Sage.
Wilson, H. (1985). *Research in nursing*. Menlo Park, CA: Addison-Wesley.

7. Exploratory Designs

Pamela J. Brink

Only recently have exploratory designs (synonymous with qualitative research) taken their place alongside descriptive and experimental designs as valid means for gaining knowledge and building theory in nursing. Beginning with Jeanne Quint Benoliel, the first graduate of the doctoral program in nursing at the University of California, San Francisco, several nurses conducting doctoral research began to use grounded theory as developed by Glaser and Strauss (1967). Their studies were presented at a series of annual western research conferences beginning in 1968. Simultaneously, in the East, particularly at Boston University, phenomenology was being introduced as a valid research approach. For many years, these exploratory designs were considered suspect by the scientific/academic community and suffered the ridicule typically encountered by new ideas. They have, however, been demonstrated to be essential designs for developing nursing knowledge. This book presents them as the first level of research design, for exploration of new research questions.

Exploratory designs have two major goals. The first is problem discovery—identifying and describing a problem area never previously studied or known. The second goal is problem definition—exploring a concept in depth in as loose and as free ranging a way as possible to arrive at a description of an experience or its meaning. Indeed, an exploratory design is also the design of choice when a problem has been identified but no literature exists on the topic. *Ethnomethodology, ethnoscience, grounded theory, qualitative research,* and *phenomenology* are all labels for designs or approaches that meet the requirements of exploratory research designs. Each type of design was developed by researchers in a different discipline to describe how they go about exploring phenomena of particular interest to them. Consequently, each differs somewhat from the others in purpose, sampling, data collection, and data analysis.

Exploratory designs use qualitative data collection methods based upon unstructured interviewing techniques, unstructured observations, unstructured available data, small samples, and a variety of forms of content analysis. They are purposefully flexible, allowing researchers to discover new phenomena or to gain new insights into known phenomena. They are also insightful, allowing for the development of new ideas, theory, and concepts. These designs enable the researcher to intuitively rearrange and make sense of the known universe, opening up an entirely new field of research in the process.

Goffman (1961) was one of the first sociologists in the United States to use the exploratory design in studying American culture; his books are now classics. Goffman made qualitative research meaningful for certain kinds of sociological questions. For example, his work on role distance resulted from watching children at play on a merry-go-round (Goffman, 1961b). His perceptive observations of their behaviors led him to propose that people distance themselves from roles that they are forced to enact but that conflict with their perceptions of themselves. This concept of role distance incorporated the notion of a "situated activity system" whereby a repetitive series of interactions is confined to a particular ongoing situation, with roles evolving that are completely separate and distinct from other roles in other situations. It was these "situated" roles from which persons became dissociated or distanced themselves.

Goffman's work on role distance was based on nonparticipant observation over time and on an intuitive analysis of what was occurring in the situation. These activities are the hallmark of exploratory studies: observing or asking about previously unexamined, everyday occurrences, trying to "tease out" the essence of what is going on. The result is an examination and subsequent explanation of the processes and procedures or rules underlying human behavior and interactions. The explanation or theory not only makes sense to anyone who has experienced something similar but also appears to have application in settings other than the one described. For example, Brink (1972) was able to use Goffman's theoretical formulation on role distance quite successfully in analyzing nurses' behaviors during daily ward rounds on a psychiatric unit in a large midwestern teaching hospital. The nurses' seemingly irrational and unprofessional behavior was interpreted as a statement of role distance for the role assigned them in that "situated activity system."

Glaser and Strauss (1967) disapproved of Goffman's published works, claiming that he focused on his incredible findings and failed to explicate his methods of collecting and analyzing data. They set about to fill this gap by describing in precise terms how to use what they termed "grounded theory." Glaser and Strauss, of course, were themselves subsequently criticized for their imprecision and accused by "hard" scientists of practicing "soft" science. The same kind of criticism has been leveled against such renowned scientists as Zborowski (1952), who made health professionals aware of cultural differences in the expression of pain; William Foote Whyte (1955), who increased knowledge with his seminal work *Street Corner Society*; and Howard Becker et al. (1961), who continued Whyte's tradition in studying medical students in *Boys in White*. Yet none of these studies has ever been seriously challenged. Quite the contrary, the insights the authors brought to their explorations have formed the groundwork for a great deal of social science theory.

The decision to use an exploratory design is frequently made when the researcher has no specific problem to study but is interested in a particular population or experience. In this situation, the exploratory design is the first step in a longitudinal research program, usually descriptive in focus. This type of exploratory research within a particular culture is common in anthropology. The research design, termed *ethnography*, encompasses both exploratory and descriptive designs, due to the longitudinal nature of the research and its emphasis upon participant observation as the basic method of data collection. In the past, anthropologists traditionally have lived in the field for at least two years in order to learn the language, find a problem, and study it in its cultural context. The works of Malinowski (Trobriand Islanders, 1922) and Radcliffe Brown (Andaman Islanders, 1922) made many persons aware of cultural relativity for the first time and created the climate for greater international understanding and respect. Current anthropologists more often enter the field with a well-defined problem and very specific objectives. Consequently, ethnography has evolved from its initial conceptualization as an exploratory descriptive design into more of a descriptive science. This outcome may reflect our increased knowledge base of other peoples and cultures.

Different types of exploratory designs are selected to achieve different outcomes. To document an experience from the perspective of the person who has lived that experience, to put into words how an experience is lived and how it feels, the design of choice is phenomenology. If the goal is to explain the antecedents, consequences, or process involved in a particular problem, then grounded theory is appropriate. Ethnomethodology or ethnographic semantics can be used to understand the cultural roles underlying a particular custom or practice. And if a clear definition of all the components of a particular phenomenon is desired, ethnoscience should be chosen. For each design, the procedures of data collection and analysis are firm and unvarying. Therefore, the researcher needs to know the desired outcome of the research in order to choose the type of qualitative design best suited to answer the question.

The underlying premise in grounded theory is that every human interaction involves a problem and a process to solve that problem. (Hutchinson, 1986, personal communication, 1987). The problem is defined through interviewing and/or participant observation, with the questions initially exploring the stages and phases of the problem. Initial interview questions might take the following form: Tell me what happened. What happened next? And then what happened? Once the problem has been isolated, questions are directed toward discovering the conditions under which the problem occurred, the precursors, the context, and the consequences.

THE BASIC EXPLORATORY DESIGN

The generic exploratory design requires the personal involvement of the investigator with a small number of people (usually fewer than 25), a small geographical or circumscribed setting (such as a hospital ward, a village, or a small interest group), repeated unstructured or semistructured interviews (usually accompanied by observations of the same subjects over time), data recorded in the form of field notes, ongoing content analysis yielding categories of mutually exclusive content, negative cases to explore further with the sample, and insights and hunches to pursue the following day.

Since the purpose of exploratory studies is to uncover something that has never been examined before, there is minimal investigator control over data. In fact, it is just the reverse: The data control the investigator. Basically, the only control the investigator has is over what is asked and what is observed. What is found then directs further questions and observations. The investigator needs to have the flexibility to "go with the flow," to challenge accepted reality and explore it for its own reality, to accept other people's rules and judgments as basic premises, to set aside prejudices and prejudgments as far as possible, and to record phenomena as they are, rather than as the researcher would like them to be.

Assumptions Underlying the Design

The following assumptions are implicit in the use of the exploratory design:

(1) The topic has not previously been studied or explored, or has not been studied from the point of view of the participant or informant.
(2) The sample has personal experience in, or knowledge about, the topic.

USE OF THE EXPLORATORY DESIGN IN NURSING

The types of studies done using this design assume the perspective of the person being interviewed or observed. The researcher is not interested in finding examples that fit an existing theory, but rather in finding examples from persons' lives that have not been heard of or imagined before. Exploratory studies examine the patient's perspective, the view from the hospital bed, the horizontal viewpoint. What is it like to face surgery? What does infant pain look like? What does privacy mean? What does health mean? What do you mean when you talked about a "good" nurse? What kinds of things have to happen to you before you seek health care? What do you expect will happen to you when you are admitted to the hospital? What will happen when you reach menopause? Puberty? What are people's expectations, in their own words; what do they think about health professionals, in their own words; and what have their experiences been in the health care system, again in their own words? What has been asked of prospective patients or clients can be asked of health professionals, of laypersons or other professionals, and of teachers and students. If you, as a researcher, want to know about any particular group, go talk to them. Ask them, from their perspective, what life is like for them. Each exploration into a particular client group adds information about the range of behaviors, beliefs, and practices of the people we nurse. We need information about people in both the healthy and the ill or traumatized state as we need to know what they want (or need) from us.

The second group of people we need to do exploratory studies on are nurses. Our major need is to document nursing interventions associated with (as well as independent of) nursing diagnosis. We need to observe nursing behaviors in interaction with patients and clients to document what nurses do with and for patients. We need to interview nurses to ask them to explain their rationale for what we observe. We need to interview nurses, and ask them to describe the patients they have known and what they have done with and for them while on the job. From these experiences we can tease out nursing action, nursing rationale, and nursing process. All of this remains exploratory.

Even if a study has previously been done that has taken the perspective of the researcher or the theorist, the same population can be studied from its own perspective. The point is to come up with new ideas, new insights, new "grounded" theories, and not to try to "fit" the data into previously delineated areas.

Long-term or longitudinal studies take an enormous amount of time, often spanning several years. In the past, many exploratory studies were not funded. They were conducted by the primary investigator with as many informants as possible, given the constraints of time and money. For example, Anderson (1987) worked as a nurse practitioner with adolescent girls at a juvenile facility. From her clinical work, she developed an interest in this population, wondering in particular what issues the girls were concerned about. Her contacts with these girls continued over a period of six years and culminated in her doctoral dissertation. Saunders (1980) interviewed newly bereaved women monthly for 13 months post-loss to explore bereavement as it was being experienced by widows whose husbands had died from different causes. Saunders obtained her subjects by searching weekly death records of the Los Angeles coroner's office. Only recently has the enormous value of studies like these been recognized by granting agencies to the extent that they have received funding.

STRENGTHS AND WEAKNESSES OF THE DESIGN

A strength of exploratory designs is the constant return to informants to verify information. Anthropological field research is usually longitudinal, with a minimum of six months spent living with the population. Phenomenology and grounded theory require a constant return to the same informants, to the same material, to continue interviewing in increasing depth. In grounded theory, for example, the investigator interviews a single informant on the selected topic, returns home, and reviews the interview, seeking gaps or missing information. The interviewer then returns to the informant and asks about the missing information. This process is repeated until the informant can provide no new information on the topic. The investigator then selects a second informant to interview and covers the same information with the second informant as has been elicited from the first. Generally, new information is gained from the second informant that must be explored in subsequent interviews. Any new information is taken back to the first informant to find out what he or she knows about it. Discrepancies in information from the two informants are noted. When no new information is obtained from the second informant, a third informant is deliberately selected and the same process is continued until no new information is elicited. This repeated return to the original informants provides verification of the information obtained, as most humans are unable to lie consistently over time. They simply cannot remember a lie as well as the truth they know, which is consistent over time.

Exploratory clinical research, or case study research, is also longitudinal, demanding a return to the same subjects again and again to ask what is happening at the moment in relation to X. The repetitive nature of the interviews and observations, over time, and on the same subjects, lends strength and credence to the exploratory study. At the same time, it discourages many individuals from conducting such research.

One weakness of this design is its lack of replicability. No single researcher can return to the same subjects, ask the same questions, and receive the same answers. Persons change their minds, their beliefs, and their positions as a result of new experiences. Therefore, the same researcher will not achieve perfect reproducibility from the same informants over time. More problematic, no other researcher can enter the same field site, find the same individuals to interview or observe, and achieve the same results. All researchers are selective in what they observe and what they report. No two humans "see" the same phenomena identically unless trained to do so, nor do they record and report identical sorts of things.

In addition, informants chosen by one researcher may not be there when the next researcher comes to study. An alternate informant may not express beliefs and values identical to those of an earlier informant. Ironically, longitudinal research mandates a relationship between researcher and informant that cannot be duplicated by another researcher, even when he or she is interviewing the same informant. The quality of that relationship makes or breaks a study, yet it is rarely reproducible.

SAMPLES

The concept of the target population is very useful in exploratory studies. The researcher strives to interview anyone who has had the experience under study. For example, if one were looking at the experience of birthing, the obvious target population would be women who have given birth. However, several details regarding the birth experience would also have to be specified. Should the sample be restricted to women who have had uneventful full-term pregnancies? Should it include women who have had spontaneous abortions, multiple births, C-sections, anomalies, or stillbirths? Should a woman's description of her experience be elicited during the event, soon after the event, or does it matter how long after the event she is queried? These questions about the target population are answered depending upon the experience under study.

A second-order question regarding the target population involves the degree to which contrasting views of the same phenomena are desired. In the birthing example, does the researcher want the experience of birthing solely from the perspective of the laboring woman, or is the perspective of her husband, birth attendant, friend, or mother also sought? Each is valuable and valid, but is it what the investigator wants? An exploratory study of birthing from the woman's perspective alone is just as valid as one eliciting all contrasting perspectives. Specification of the desired perspective is critical to all definitions of the target population.

Exploratory design calls for small samples that are chosen through a deliberative process to represent the desired perspective. (Grounded theorists call this *theoretical sampling,* as the sample must be theoretically relevant to the question.) For this reason samples are usually purposive. The rationale for selection of informants depends upon the purpose of the research. If the purpose is to discover a problem, then the target population is frequently selected on the basis of personal interest of the researcher. Aamodt (1981) selected a Norwegian community in the Midwest because her relatives lived there; Ragucci (1981) selected an Italian neighborhood in Boston because she was living in Boston and was herself Italian-American. Personal relationships also frequently provide entry to the field site or the target population. An acquaintance can introduce the researcher around, making access to the population easier and allaying suspicions about the researcher's intentions.

METHODS OF DATA COLLECTION

Exploratory designs call for unstructured data collection methods, usually participant observation with interviewing. Many quantitative researchers have difficulty with exploratory studies because of their flexible data collection procedures and lack of specificity. Since the point of the research is to get at the desired information in the best or most efficient way possible, a trial-and-error approach to what works, with whom, and when, is required. Because not every human understands a question in exactly the same way, a flexible approach helps the researcher to find the best question for a given individual to understand and answer. Here are some examples based upon Spradley and McCurdy (1972):

- *Grand tour questions* (setting the tone for the interview or questionnaire): "I would like you to tell me about the last experience you had with a person you thought was a 'problem patient.' "
- *Contrast or comparative questions:* "Tell me what you think are the differences between men and women in relation to their ability to be successful weight losers. In what way do you think they are similar?"

- *Inclusive questions:* ''What kinds of studies are research studies?'' Or, ''If you were to define and give examples of qualitative nursing research, what studies would you cite?''
- *Exclusive questions:* ''If you were to develop a new community program in eldercare, who would not be eligible?'' Or, ''What kinds of research would you say are not examples of qualitative nursing research?''

Perhaps the most important element of exploratory research is not the questions that are asked per se, but the interview itself. Because analysis is based upon the interview in its entirety, and not on each specific question, the interviewer's approach to the interview is of paramount importance. In their book on the cultural experience, Spradley and McCurdy (1972) talk about the ''grand tour question,'' an opening gambit for finding out ''what's going on here.'' The grand tour question sets the tone, opens the discussion, and lets everyone know what the interview is about. Since not everyone would know how to answer the question, What's going on here? without some preliminary information, it is necessary for the investigator to explain about the topic of the research. Simply approaching an informant abruptly and asking ''Tell me all about your birthing experience,'' might elicit some very odd answers. Instead, the investigator tells the informants what is being studied and why, what aroused the investigator's interest in the topic or area, and so on. In this way, the investigator ''primes the pump,'' so to speak. Informants may be cued in by a simple statement, such as ''Ever since I gave birth to my first child, I have wondered if other women have gone through the same feelings I have had. So I decided I'd like to ask other women about their experiences with birth.''

Some investigators begin not by asking questions, but rather by ''entering the field'' and ''getting a feel for'' the area. Anderson (1987) would not have succeeded with the girls at the juvenile facility if she had begun by asking direct questions, because they would not have trusted her. Being an employee in the facility, however, she had a legitimate reason to interact with the girls, and spent a great deal of time with them on the unit prior to developing her research questions. Anderson's approach was not unlike the approach of anthropologists who enter a Pacific island community or an African village for an extended period of time, getting a feel for the place, meeting people, finding the post office and grocery store, and generally watching everyone to find out who's who and what's going on. Only later, when widespread familiarity has been established, does the investigator begin asking direct, but unstructured, questions in formal interviews. Prior to that time, all interviews could be considered informal conversations, which nevertheless provide a great deal of data about the field site and the population.

Two other, perhaps more familiar, examples of the unstructured interview are the clinical interview and the mental status examination. The goal of these interviews is to assess the level of functioning of the client. Although the clinician has in mind an outline of the facts needed to achieve the goal, in neither case does he or she rely on a predetermined set of questions or a predetermined ordering of questions. Although these interviews are completely unstructured, the inherent validity or reliability of the obtained data are not questioned in clinical practice. Although errors can occur in eliciting information from an informant, these errors are just as possible with a standardized or structured questionnaire.

DATA ANALYSIS

Data analysis in exploratory research, like data collection, requires a fluid, flexible, somewhat intuitive interaction, this time between the investigator and the data. Essentially, the investigator "lives with" the data, reading and rereading field notes on a daily or frequent basis and deciding what has been learned so far, what is puzzling, what is unanswered, and what does not fit. The investigator takes notes, writes self-reminders about what is wanted (a technique called "memoing"; see Chapter 8), and prepares for the next interaction with informants. New questions may be written out in advance, old questions may be asked again, or an observation might be planned. This material provides the basis for new fieldwork and subsequent field notes, which themselves are analyzed in exactly the same way. This process of interaction between data collection and analysis continues throughout the field experience or the periods of data collection.

Because analysis, including the development of hunches and insights, requires the personal involvement of the investigator with the data, no one but the investigator can be involved in the process. There is simply no room for a research assistant at this stage of analysis. The analysis itself is a holistic examination of all collected data at the same time. Exploratory analysis thus contrasts with descriptive analysis, in which each individual's responses to questions are examined separately.

Several analytic methods can be used in exploratory studies, depending upon the specific type of design: Constant comparison and saturation of categories, yielding a theoretical model, is used in grounded theory (Glaser & Strauss, 1967); componential analysis, yielding a taxonomy of terms, is used in ethnomethodology (Spradley & McCurdy, 1972); thematic analysis, yielding the essence of the lived experience is used in phenomenology (Van Manen, 1984); and reading participant observation field notes over and over in their totality to derive a descriptive distillation of the meaning of the material is used in analytic induction (Wilson, 1985). The analysis process sifts through the information, within context, to arrive at a description that makes sense to both those who have lived the experience and those who have no prior knowledge of the concept or content.

Since all data take the form of words, sentences, and paragraphs, the smallest unit of analysis is the single word or concept, which can be treated as a nominal scale item. As in semantic analysis, however, it is possible to categorize all terms into mutually exclusive saturated categories that, taken together, describe the concept in its entirety. Content analysis therefore involves making decisions about the categories of content and assigning code numbers or code labels to those categories. The entire text of data is then completely coded. Every bit of collected information can be coded, using as many categories as needed. Consider, for example, an interview in which an informant describes a series of steps involved in making pasta. Each sentence may include material on the recipe, the carbohydrate content, the color, texture, weight, density, or taste of the pasta, and consequently may be coded under more than one category. These codes are a simple means of differentiating content for filing or retrieval purposes and are immensely useful in computer analysis of data using a search feature. If any form of structured analysis is wanted, such as the number of times an item was mentioned or the number of people who mentioned the item, availability of a computer search is important. When the accumulated data are extensive, this form of analysis becomes critical.

HUMAN SUBJECTS ISSUES

As with any other research, the principal investigator must be aware of the need for informed consent, confidentiality, and anonymity. However, the three major problems involving ethics in human research (invasion of privacy, withholding benefits, and coercion to participate) are not all problematic in exploratory research. Invasion of privacy can be a concern in exploratory studies, particularly when the subjects are patients or clients and the researcher is a professional within the system. Withholding benefits, associated primarily with experimental research, does not concern the exploratory researcher, who may not know what the benefits might be until the study is over. Institutional review panels, however, being particularly concerned with cost-benefit ratios, sometimes question exploratory research precisely because the investigator cannot specify the possible benefit of the research in advance or predict the outcome prior to data collection. Whenever benefits cannot be specified, they are considered to be outweighed by the risks. This is one reason the "expedited review" has been developed for social science research. If an investigator can document that the informants will be able to understand the research and can discontinue participation at any time, then just talking to the investigator is not considered a major risk.

The investigator also needs to document the means by which confidentiality and anonymity will be established and maintained. How the investigator explains to informants what will happen to their stories or interviews, and whether or not their names, stories, and location will be made public is critical. If audio- or videotapes are to be made of the subjects, what will happen to these tapes? Because much exploratory research yields new information, handling of data, particularly from fieldwork in foreign countries, can have political implications. Protection of the subject is paramount, even to the extent of destroying research records if necessary.

THE RESEARCH PROPOSAL

Exploratory research studies are not funded as frequently as other types of designs, because they do not lend themselves to detailed proposals. (See Tripp-Reimer & Cohen, 1989, for a more detailed description of grant proposal writing.) The major budgetary items in exploratory studies involve travel for interviews, transcription of taped or filmed interviews, and salaries. Nevertheless, investigators submitting grant proposals need to recognize several problems they are likely to encounter.

First, exploratory research is often conducted by the investigator alone simply because exploratory researchers prefer to interact with the data and answer the questions themselves. Consequently, few exploratory researchers have research assistants to help them with data collection. Research assistance, whether for data collection, data analysis, or computer analysis, increases the size of a grant proposal budget. More recently, among grounded theorists particularly, teams of researchers are working together to study a single problem area. Field research in foreign countries or well-demarcated communities is usually conducted using field teams, but, again, the predominant form is the single researcher going to the field and hiring informants there.

An even more difficult problem encountered in grant writing is how to justify funding a proposal that has no question or hypothesis. How does a review panel determine the importance of a project if the investigator cannot specify what is being studied? Therefore, the first task of the researcher is to "declare" a problem area within which exploration will be conducted. This problem area will of necessity be a broad one, in order to allow the latitude necessary for later formulation of a valid question. But granting agencies usually require a defined problem that is tied to a literature base, and usually to some theory. Since most exploratory researchers cannot specify the problem this neatly at the outset, they often cannot obtain grants at this stage of the research. The Center for Nursing Research now has more qualitative researchers as members of its scientific panel who understand the problems of grant writing for qualitative methods. They recommend that the researcher "walk" the review committee through the proposed steps in the process, talk about the literature that was reviewed and what was found, provide the panel with an understanding of why this research is different from the current literature (other than in its method), and, finally, give the panel an idea of the kind of outcome desired, whether in the form of a table, a short descriptive paragraph, or a concept.

The third area that causes major problems in proposal writing is the sample. Frequently, exploratory researchers have no idea what the size of the sample will be at the beginning of the study, since the size of the sample is dictated by the comprehensiveness of the data to be collected. Exploratory researchers frequently find more and more persons to interview, until they have "saturated their categories" (Glaser & Strauss, 1967; Hutchinson, 1986) or until nothing new is being added to the data base. For this reason, specifying sample size at the outset is problematic. Review panels, which generally need specificity and closure, require investigators to make an educated guess at the sample size. Is it possible to complete the task with 10 persons or 25? Might it take 50? The researcher must pick a reasonable number or specify a time frame for data collection to be devoted to the project. For instance, "the data will be collected on a minimum of 10 persons over a period of six months." Or, "a maximum of 25 subjects will be interviewed over a period of six months."

Most exploratory designs pose problems for reliability. The standard methods of establishing reliability would require something like test-retest reliability of the research subjects, or having another researcher interview the same or similar informants and achieve the same results. As explained earlier, neither of these is likely to be possible. Therefore, the research proposal should address those forms of reliability that can be used in qualitative data collection (see Brink, 1989).

Reliability is primarily determined by the investigator's use of alternate-form questions while interviewing informants, or by the use of two observers (interrater reliability) during initial observations. (In this case the second observer is not a member of a research team but is called in on an ad hoc basis to provide a reliability check.) Exploratory researchers always ask the same questions in a variety of ways in order to ensure that the answers given by the informants are indeed similar. Since many exploratory researchers also interview the same informant several times on the same topic, alternate-form questions become built into the method of data collection. In other words, repeating questions to the same subject on the same topic over time provides a form of test-retest reliability. The questions used to monitor test-retest reliability are critical. If the question reflects changes over time, test-retest is not possible. If the question used is a point of past fact, the answer should be the same each time. How alternate-form reliability will be used should be described in detail. Brink (1989), Brink and Wood (1988), Polit and Hungler (1987), and Selltiz et al. (1981) can be cited as references.

Unelaborated descriptions of methodology are also problematic in proposals for exploratory studies. Because there are no standardized instruments, the procedures for data collection need to be specified in as much detail as possible. The review panel needs to know precisely how data will be collected from each informant and what will be done if enough information is not obtained from that person. The researcher should try to give the review panel all the information they need to make a clear recommendation. This information might include an example of an interview, a description of what will be looked for, a chart depicting use of available data, a poem, a letter, an oral history— whatever will be used.

Although exploratory studies are inherently nonreplicable, few qualitative researchers question their validity (Pelto & Pelto, 1978); review panels, however, usually do. The type of validation sought is very important to the success of a grant proposal. Most exploratory research studies have pragmatic or concurrent validation (Brink, 1989; Brink & Wood, 1988; Polit & Hungler, 1987; Selltiz et al., 1981) "built into the design," since they use more than one method of data collection. Usually interviewing is accompanied by observation or available data or both. In this way data are "triangulated" (Sohier, 1989) or validated by alternate methods, just as the informant is deemed reliable through the use of alternate forms of questions. Unlike quantitative studies, in which concurrent validation is achieved through the use of another, previously validated, instrument, no previously validated instrument exists in exploratory studies. Therefore, utilizing different methods of data collection is extremely important in establishing the validity of the data. For example, Dean and Whyte (1969) discuss the interesting issue of how a researcher knows if the informant is telling the truth.

During a participant observation study on an Indian reservation, Brink (1969) interviewed mothers about their child-rearing habits. When one mother was asked, "What do you do when your baby cries?" she replied, "I pick him up." However, as the interviewer sat with this mother in her front room, her toddler crawled over, pulled himself up on her knee and hit his head on a table. Although he began to scream and cry, the mother ignored him. She did not pick him up and hold him in her lap until he tugged at her clothing. Had the investigator not observed this incident, the answer to her question would have been recorded as the mother gave it. This example demonstrates the difficulty of obtaining valid self-report data without some form of alternative or substantiating information.

Finally, the fluid and unstructured sample and methodology make the data analysis section of a proposal difficult. Review panels understand content analysis (Krippendorf, 1980), but they may not understand "musing," or "thematic analysis," or a "lived experience" (see Chapter 8). Again, the researcher must try to describe for the panel what he or she would do with an interview, an observation, or a poem. If the analysis and data collection plans allow it, the researcher can label a single section of the proposal "Methods and Analysis" and can discuss them simultaneously. This is particularly useful for grounded theory and phenomenology. The use of constant comparison requires analysis of each interview as it compares with preceding interviews in order for the researcher to decide how to interview the next informant. Such approaches must be described in detail.

A major problem with exploratory research proposals is their mixing of grounded theory with phenomenology. If the researcher uses grounded theory in data collection and sampling, then constant comparison should be used in data analysis. Grounded theory resources should be referenced for grounded theory approaches. A phenomenological study is at a disadvantage when mixed with grounded theory approaches. *Thematic analysis, musings,* and *bracketing* are all phenomenological terms, and their use should be limited to proposals for studies using that approach. Again, because each approach is very different, documentation is very important.

CRITIQUE OF EXPLORATORY DESIGNS

When critiquing an exploratory study, one should look for the name of the design somewhere in the paper. If a design is named, then the paper must meet the design criteria. For example, if an author states that the design is grounded theory, one should look for theoretical sampling, constant comparisons, and the delineation of a core variable underlying the theory. The final theoretical outcome should be some type of basic psychological or interactional process that forms the central theme of the paper (Hutchinson, 1986, p. 119). If these criteria are not met, the paper may be critiqued as a generic exploratory study. The author should also be informed of the error.

An article based upon phenomenology will not include much explication of the method. Like historical research, the findings are considered to be more important than the techniques and procedures used to derive the description. The report may be written in a variety of ways, and it is up to the reader to decide whether it is complete and comprehensive according to the method of presentation. Since phenomenology is essentially an example composed of other examples, the number of questions remaining after reading the example gives an indication of the author's success in describing the phenomena or the lived experience. Van Manen (1984, pp. 26-27) has stated that a phenomenological report can be written thematically, analytically, exemplicatively, existentially, or exegetically (organized in the form of a dialogue with another phenomenological writer). Any of these approaches is acceptable in a phenomenological study.

If an author uses qualitative methods in a generic exploratory design, the reader should look for the development of the problem; a literature review that supports the question, the methods, and the sample; evidence of the reliability and validity of the researcher as the research instrument; and content analysis yielding a basic listing of the components of the report. These elements are frequently more brief than they would be in an experimental design, since the bulk of the report will focus upon the findings. No section should be missing, however, and all sections should be relevant to the findings. The reader should look for any missing or mismatched parts, such as failure to describe the sample, use of structured data collection instruments, or attempts at enumeration. The findings should always describe a process, a phenomenon, or a new theoretical formulation. Again, the reader should have little sense of incompleteness or unanswered questions. If this exists, the article needs rewriting.

Particular caution is necessary when evaluating a researcher's sample. In Rosenhahn's classic paper, "On Being Sane in Insane Places" (1976), it is difficult to determine if the eight fieldworkers were the sample or if the eight hospital wards were the intended sample. In reality, however, it makes no difference. The outcome of the research remains the same—namely, the staff were unable to differentiate between "planted pseudopatients" and regular patients. Rosenhahn was, on the basis of this study, able to propose a theory of "labeling" to describe how health professionals (like others) often interact with labels and stereotypes rather than with individuals.

SUMMARY

Essential features of the exploratory design are as follows:

(1) problem discovery or problem definition as the research goal
(2) small purposive or theoretical samples of 25 or fewer
(3) longitudinal rather than cross-sectional data collection
(4) multiple interviews over time on the same subject, as opposed to one-shot interviews
(5) repeated measures on the same subject
(6) unstructured data collection techniques and procedures
(7) continuous analysis of data, with return to subjects for verification
(8) formulation of a new concept, definition, explanation, or theory, or description of a process or experience

REFERENCES

Anderson, N. L. (1987). *Doing time and making choices: The anthropology of pregnancy resolution decisions in juvenile detention.* Unpublished doctoral dissertation, University of California, Los Angeles.

Becker, H. S., et al. (1961). *Boys in white.* Chicago: University of Chicago Press.

Brink, P. J. (1969). *The northern Paiute.* Unpublished doctoral dissertation, Boston University.

Brink, P. J. (1972). Role distance: A maneuver in nursing. *Nursing Forum, 11*(3), 323-332.

Brink, P. J. (1989). Issues in reliability and validity. In J. M. Morse (Ed.), *Qualitative nursing research: A contemporary dialogue* (pp. 139-154). Rockville, MD: Aspen.

Brink, P. J., & Wood, M. J. (1988). *Basic steps in planning nursing research: From question to proposal* (3rd ed.). Boston: Jones & Bartlett.

Dean, J. P., & Whyte, W. F. (1969). How do you know if the informant is telling the truth? In G. J. McCall & J. L. Simmons (Eds.), *Issues in participation observation: A text and reader* (pp. 105-115). Reading, MA: Addison-Wesley.

Glaser, B. G., & Strauss, A. (1967). *The discovery of grounded theory: Strategies for qualitative research.* New York: Aldine-Atherton.

Goffman, E. (1961a). *Asylums.* Garden City, NY: Doubleday.

Goffman, E. (1961b). *Encounters: Two studies in the sociology of interaction.* Indianapolis: Bobbs-Merrill.

Goffman, E. (1963). *Stigma: Notes on the management of spoiled identity.* Englewood Cliffs, NJ: Prentice-Hall.

Hutchinson, S. (1986). Grounded theory: The method. In P. L.Munhall & C. J. Oiler (Eds.), *Nursing research: A qualitative perspective* (pp. 111-130). Norwalk, CT: Appleton-Century-Crofts.

Krippendorf, K. (1980). *Content analysis: An introduction to its methodology*. Beverly Hills, CA: Sage.

Munhall, P. L., & Oiler, C. J. (Eds.). (1986). *Nursing research: A qualitative perspective*. Norwalk, CT: Appleton-Century-Crofts.

Pelto, P. J., & Pelto, G. H. (1978). *Anthropological research: The structure of inquiry* (2nd ed.). Cambridge: Cambridge University Press.

Polit, D. F., & Hungler, B. P. (1987). *Nursing research*. Philadelphia: J. B. Lippincott.

Ragucci, A. (1981). Italian Americans. In A. Harwood (Ed.), *Ethnicity and medical care* (pp. 211-263). Cambridge, MA: Harvard University Press.

Rosenhahn, D. L. (1976). On being sane in insane places. In P. J. Brink (Ed.), *Transcultural nursing: A book of readings* (pp. 175-197). Englewood Cliffs, NJ: Prentice-Hall.

Saunders, J. (1981). A process of bereavement resolution: Uncoupled identity. *Western Journal of Nursing Research, 3*, 319-336.

Selltiz, C., Wrightsman, L. S., & Cook, S. W. (1981). *Research methods in social relations* (4th ed.). New York: Holt, Rinehart & Winston.

Sohier, R. (1989). Multiple triangulation and contemporary nursing research. *Western Journal of Nursing Research, 10*, 732-742.

Spradley, J. P., & McGurdy, D. W. (1972). *The cultural experience: Ethnography in complex society*. Chicago: Science Research Associates.

Swanson-Kauffman, K. M. (1986, April). A combined qualitative methodology for nursing research. *Advances in Nursing Science*, pp. 58-69.

Tripp-Reimer, T., & Cohen, M. Z. (1989). Funding strategies for qualitative research. In J.M. Morse (Ed.), *Qualitative nursing research: A contemporary dialogue* (pp. 209-220). Rockville, MD: Aspen.

Van Manen, M. (1984). *"Doing" phenomenological research and writing: An introduction* (Monograph No. 7). Alberta: University of Alberta, Faculty of Education, Department of Secondary Education.

Whyte, W. F. (1955). *Street corner society: The social structure of an Italian slum*. Chicago: University of Chicago Press.

Wilson, H. (1985). *Research in nursing*. Menlo Park, CA: Addison-Wesley.

Zborowski, M. (1952). Cultural components in response to pain. *Journal of Social Issues, 8*, 16-30.

8. Qualitative Designs

Patricia L. Munhall

A growing enthusiasm and interest in qualitative research designs has broadened the research perspective of nurse researchers today. Lively discussions and enlightening critiques are a part of the evolving research paradigm for nursing (see Morse, 1989). The prevalent qualitative research methods that nurse researchers seem most interested in are phenomenology, grounded theory, ethnography, history, case studies, and analytic philosophy. Discussions of these methods can be found in texts by Leininger (1985), Field and Morse (1985), Munhall and Oiler (1986), Parse, Coyne, and Smith (1985), Swanson and Chenitz (1986), and Morse (1989).

Qualitative research methods have been explained by Benoliel (1984)

> as modes of systematic inquiry concerned with understanding human beings and the nature of their transactions with themselves and with their surroundings. (p. 3)

She further states:

> Qualitative approaches in science are distinct modes of inquiry oriented toward understanding the unique nature of human thoughts, behaviors, negotiations and institutions under different sets of historical and environmental circumstances. (p. 7)

Field and Morse (1985) write:

> Qualitative methods should be used when there is little known about a domain, when the investigator suspects that the present knowledge

or theories may be biased or when the research question pertains to understanding or describing a particular phenomenon or event about which little is known. (p. 11)

Wilson (1985) points to the nonqualitative aspects of qualitative research and posits:

> Qualitative analysis is the nonnumerical organization and interpretation of data in order to discover patterns, themes, forms and qualities found in field notes, interview transcripts, open-ended questionnaires, journals and diaries. (p. 397)

Leininger (1985) offers this conception:

> The qualitative type of research refers to the methods and techniques of observing, documenting, analyzing and interpreting attributes, patterns, characteristics and meanings of specific, contextual or gestaltic features of phenomena under study. (p. 5)

This chapter focuses on two qualitative designs or the methods of phenomenology and grounded theory. The intention is to introduce the nurse researcher to some of the underlying ideas and assumptions of qualitative research. The chapter is an overview, and as such does not answer as many questions as it raises. In that spirit, references are provided for those readers who may find their nursing research interests philosophically compatible with qualitative research methods and who are spurred on to further discovery.

QUALITATIVE DESIGN: A BEGINNING[1]

A person or situation presents interests, problems, or questions, and we can often respond in one of two ways. We can respond from extrapolation and hunches about what is known or assumed about the phenomenon, or we can suspend preconceptions or inferences and say, "I'm not sure about that," "I don't know about that," or "There's virtually nothing known about that." The first approach leads to deduction, the latter to induction. The first response lends itself to traditional hypothesis testing and deduction from existing theory; the second response lends itself to going out and finding out what's going on and leads to theory development.

For example, consider the question, What's it like being divorced? A deductive approach to this question would be to arrive at some hunches from the literature on divorce and the family, from existing role theory, from developmental theory, from psychology, and so on. The hunches would become hypotheses, linking some variables found in the literature to, in this instance, divorce. They would be, as called for, directional, and might have as dependent variables increased role stress, role conflict, or role ambiguity. There may be increased life satisfaction, increased sense of generativity, or decreased interaction with old friends. The variables deduced from the literature could be endless. Regardless, the researcher would test hypotheses using, say, a quasi-experimental or correlational design to support or refute hypotheses based on a statistical level of significance. The answer to the question, then, is based primarily on what can be deduced from what is already known.

In contrast, the answer to the question can be approached from a qualitative perspective. This is particularly appropriate when there have been rapid sociological changes, so that if theory does exist, it may be outdated and no longer relevant. With a qualitative design, the answer may be obtained by asking people the question in a direct way and/or by spending time observing and interacting with people who are divorced. Interviewing people, observing people, and, perhaps, in this case, asking people to keep diaries or other written records would all yield fresh authentic data. Questions that lend themselves to qualitative approaches might start with "What's going on here?" "How does it feel to be . . . ?" "What does the experience mean?" or "What's it like to be . . . ?"

With a qualitative design, we are seeking to discover knowledge, to develop or reformulate theory from the authentic source. We are looking at the whole within context.

The interest in qualitative designs is directed toward discovering or uncovering new insights, meanings, and understandings. The research is often serendipitous, leads often to wonderment, and requires from the researcher an ability to remain flexible. Other assumptions that should be considered concerning qualitative designs include the following:

(1) There may be a current theory about the subject we wish to investigate, but what is known may now be out of contemporary context. Answers to the question, What's it like being divorced? differ dramatically from

one generation to another. Theories need to be revised in light of societal changes, other new discoveries, and human evolution. Theory is culturally and time bounded. As culture "advances" and time progresses, different descriptions and explanations are critical to accurate understanding.

(2) Nursing has advanced a philosophy that embraces the whole of the human condition. We profess to values that include respect for all individuals and their cultural interpretations of meaning in experience and events. Following from this is an emphasis on self-determination and autonomy. A qualitative perspective then becomes essential from the philosophical perspective of nursing not only as a research design, but for actual implementation of a holistic, empathic, individualized delivery of nursing care. In the discussion below of phenomenology as a design for research, we will see that a broad question could be asked, such as, What is the lived experience of being divorced about? An exploratory, open, theory-suspended approach actualizes the belief that the individual interprets his or her own experiences and gives meaning to them.

(3) With many qualitative designs, there is an attempted suspension or bracketing out of what we have already come to believe, suspect, or assume. Qualitative designs yield new understanding and insights.

(4) Qualitative designs are needed in current theory formulation and reformulation to assess the extent to which gender biases have influenced our view of the world and have established norms and standards that may be inappropriately generalized. Sex bias research results in asymmetry of findings, role stereotyping (parent = mother), failure to address sex as a variable whether a subject variable or a stimulus variable, and a general devaluation of women's interpretation modes and epistemological interests. There is a growing recognition of the need to reexamine and perhaps reconstruct theories so that gender, class, and ethnic background are recognized outright. Qualitative designs are critical to this pursuit.

When to Use Qualitative Designs

Qualitative designs are appropriate

(1) when virtually nothing seems known about a topic or phenomenon;
(2) when what seems to be known or believed somehow does not seem accurate (intuiting), prompting
   (a) hunches about inconsistencies,
   (b) hunches about biases,
   (c) hunches that time has changed what is believed, or
   (d) hunches about ineffective approaches;
(3) when feelings arise such as
   (a) "something doesn't ring true,"

(b) "that's not real life," or

(c) "something's going on here and I'm not quite sure what it is"; or

(4) when the researcher wonders what it would feel like to experience something he or she knows nothing about.

As mentioned, a researcher might want to explore the design itself, taking on the question, What's the lived experience of doing a qualitative design like? (Hutchinson, 1985, gives a good description of that process.) An important dimension to the process is to become comfortable with the philosophical and ethical underpinnings of qualitative designs (see Field & Morse, 1985; Leininger, 1985; Munhall & Oiler, 1986; Parse et al., 1985; Swanson & Chenitz, 1986).

PHENOMENOLOGY AS METHOD

Omery (1983) notes that "most researchers in the social sciences who have advocated or implemented the phenomenological method have been inspired by it, rather than directly apply steps" (p. 53). This is a critical point to remember when defending a departure from some lockstep designs. The point here illustrates the philosophy/design juncture. The philosophy is open, interpretive, and individualistic. Designs with prescribed steps in themselves are prescriptive and give direction to the lived experience of doing phenomenology as interpreted by a phenomenological philosopher or researcher. In this sense, they contradict the philosophy. The researcher should recognize that such contradictions are part of the lived experience of doing phenomenology and, accepting that, move on, remembering the theme of "being inspired" rather than of strictly applying steps.

Regardless, for most of us, a "where to begin" and a "how to do it" frame our thinking and help us actualize the concepts and beliefs underpinning the method. The question of how to gain access to lived experience then is answered by many philosophers and social scientists. Among those who have advanced a particular method are Giorgi, VanKaam, Spiegelberg, Colaizzi, Merleau-Ponty, and the Utrecht school (method) as practiced by Martinus Langveld. The researcher contemplating a particular phenomenological method should consult the work of these authors, and should look at various studies using these methods; however, he or she should remember that to be faithfully phenomenological, a study should not necessarily be structured by a linear design. The experience itself will often provide the direction.

In the discussions of the two studies that follow, we can see how two nurse researchers have been inspired by phenomenological philosophy. Oiler (1982, 1983) uses Spiegelberg's phenomenological method to guide her through the task of exploring a phenomenological perspective in nursing, and Sauer's (1985) study advances her own interpretation of a phenomenological method. Both demonstrate qualitative designs in that both ask questions concerning phenomena about which virtually nothing is known in nursing—Oiler asks what a phenomenological perspective in nursing is like, and Sauer asks about what it is like having a child later in life than is the cultural norm.

Oiler and Spiegelberg

In Oiler's "The Phenomenological Approach in Nursing Research" (1982), nurses' expression in the art form of poetry are utilized to examine nursing reality. The "lived experience" of the nurse is a critical dimension in nursing practice, in that nurses' ideas about that reality continuously inform and dirct nursing practice, education, and reality. Oiler (1982) notes:

> Nurse poets help us to see nursing reality by disrupting our customary way of referring to it with technical language. In the poetic form, the nursing situation is seen from a different vantage point. Poetic expression enlarges our view, giving us an opportunity to know about nursing experience in a different way. (p. 121)

The aims of the study were (1) to examine the concept of subjectivity in the nursing literature, (2) to describe a phenomenological perspective in nursing, and (3) to contribute to a clarification of lived experience. Spiegelberg's method of phenomenology inspired Oiler's exploration into phenomenology and demonstrates the underlying concepts of this philosophical perspective on reality.

One Phenomenological Method

Spiegelberg's (1976) method of doing phenomenology was utilized as a guideline. The essential operations are briefly described here, and the same steps are presented in a second format.

(1) *Bracketing*: This is a process by which the researcher attempts to be, to the extent possible, free of bias, working to recognize bias and "control" for it. To see lived experience, one must suspend and lay aside what one thinks one already knows about it. Since the researcher wishes to recognize what it is, he or she thinks about an experience and then brackets or suspends it—a literature review at this point would only give the researcher more to bracket out. The more unknown the subject is, the less bracketing is necessary. The researcher might write a description of everything he or she knows or believes about the topic of exploration and then set it aside.

(2) *Intuiting*: Here the researcher becomes absorbed in the phenomenon, looking at it fresh, without layering it with what he or she has bracketed out. Concentration is very important here, as the involvement is very intense.

(3) *Analyzing*: At this point the researcher compares and contrasts descriptions of the phenomenon under study. This allows for identification of recurring themes and interrelationships.

(4) *Describing*: This is the final step for the researcher: communciating to others what he or she has found. This is the actual communication of phenomenological seeing.

For Spiegelberg, these steps are for the purpose of investigating particular phenomena, investigating general essences, and apprehending essential relationships among essences.

Procedures in Oiler's Study

Nursing journals published over the past ten years were reviewed for poems authored by nurses. During a three-month period, 58 poems were read and reread. This was a "dwelling with" period, in which the researcher attempted to lay aside what she might write in poetry or another aesthetic form, instead imaginatively and intuitively assuming another's point of view. This allowed for the emergence of recurring themes, which then enabled description of particular phenomena, general essences, and essential relationshps among essences. The value and opportunities of aesthetic expressions for understanding lived experience cannot be overstated.

With qualitative designs in particular, every avenue of access to awareness should be looked at and dwelled with. In the process of dwelling with the language of poetry, Oiler (1980) gained access to nurses' lived realities, and because she attempted to bracket out what

she knew about the world, she allowed different awarenesses to surface. The researcher attempted to suspend her preconceptions and/or
conceptions and look at experience fresh. From such newly gleaned
awarenesses descriptive theory can emerge.

Descriptions

In the examination of selected poems, Oiler discovered the intensity
of nurses' emotional responses to nurse-client situations. We learn of
this part of nurse valuing—the determination to explicate the meaning of caring in the nursing situation. We learn that such human expression brings meaning to existence. Oiler moves beyond technical
language and meanings that objectify the world, which, as Zbilut (1977)
notes, leave much of nursing experience in silence.

Returning to Spiegelberg's three purposes (investigating phenomena,
general essences, and essential relationships among essences), let us
review what has been described.

Themes, Essences, and Interrelationships

Oiler's work reveals many themes, essences, and interrelationships:

(1) nurses feeling angry and frustrated; awareness of obstructed pursuit;
    interrelationship with feminist theory development
(2) nurses as nurturers, and as surrogate and real mothers; interrelation-
    ships of dependence and independence; letting go, ambivalence, and
    changing roles
(3) nurses struggling with the risks of closeness, pain of separation, tensions
    between person and role, and a need to integrate personal history more
    adequately through the role
(4) nurses' awareness of the meaning of patients' circumstances in the con-
    text of the life cycle

Thus this study reveals themes, essences, and interrelationships that
should command our attention. The use of a qualitative design in this
instance allows us to come closer to the experience of nursing. Implications from the descriptions are critical to the nursing profession, to
nurses as individuals, and to the recipients of nursing care. One can
imagine the consequences, or perhaps we already know the consequences, of not attending to these responses. A qualitative design such
as this enables us to answer the question, What's going on here? when

perhaps the consequences are already being felt as problems. Such consequences of the above essences and theories might include attrition, low morale, burnout, and the like. The findings from this study enable an enlightened view of the experience and thus enable knowledgeable and relevant intervention. Thus Oiler has accomplished her aims of examining the concept of subjectivity in nursing literature, describing a phenomenological perspective, and contributing to the clarification of lived experience.

Sauer and Her Own Phenomenological Method

Sauer (1985) related that the phenomenological method with which she is most familiar is the Utrecht school method as taught and practiced by Martinus Langveld of the Netherlands. In this interpretation of method, the concept of transformation is critical and is referred to as the "validity of their (phenomenologists') claims to knowledge." Sauer then goes on to use Reinharz's (1983) five steps of phenomenological transformation to underpin the advancement of her "own" method. Sauer's personal interpretation concurs with Omery's (1983) statement that this phenomenological method is often interpreted within the philosophy rather than by applying a specific set of steps.

- *First transformation*: A person's experience is transformed into actions and language that become available to him or her by special interaction with the phenomenological researcher.
- *Second transformation*: The researcher transforms what is heard into an understanding of the original experience.
- *Third transformation*: The researcher attempts to capture the essence of the original experience by clarifying conceptual categories.
- *Fourth transformation*: These conceptual categories are transformed into some type of written or visual description that attempts to capture the experience the person has spoken about.
- *Fifth transformation*: This written or visual description clarifies for the recipients of the description the phenomenon under investigation.

The Aim of the Study

Sauer (1985) states that the aim of her study was to "clearly understand a poorly delineated phase in the life cycle of a modern woman, that is, the timing of childbearing" (p. 98). Specifically, the study focused on couples planning to have their first child later in life than is usual in their culture. The phenomenological method, as interpreted by Sauer, was carried out in the following steps:

(1) Interviews were conducted with three couples as they lived through the last three months of a delayed pregnancy and the first three months of parenthood. Two additional women were interviewed during the last month of pregnancy. Sauer also used literature, in the form of Phyllis Chesler's book, *With Child: A Diary of Motherhood* (1979). In the spirit of bracketing, Sauer delayed using some of her own and her husband's experience when, toward the end of this study, she herself became pregnant.

(2) *First transformation:* Interviews took place in the informants' homes, with the goal of creating a setting that would make possible near natural conversation. Sauer recorded notes, and, in an effort to ensure accuracy of her recordings, gave informants transcriptions of their interviews. Thus the informants had the opportunity to validate that the materials expressed what they meant to say.

(3) *Classification of conceptual categories:* Sauer describes the overwhelming process of analyzing the dialogues and separating out themes for each informant. With themes identified for each informant, variations in themes could be selected out. In reporting the data, the headings "Forms" (themes) and "Variations" were used so that ground structure or clarifying conceptual categories could be identified. For example, the identification of a conceptual category of "planned, orderly lives" was advanced as one of the ground structures of the lived experiences of delayed parenthood for women.

(4) *Description and essences:* The meaningfulness of transition to delayed parenthood becomes more comprehensible when viewed from this conceptual framework of "planned, orderly lives." Sauer expands our understanding of this experience and its ramifications when she reminds us that with planning comes a sense of control. She notes that these individuals actually "planned" their pregnancies and then revealed "shock, surprise, and disbelief" at what they found to be an uncontrollable situation.

The foregoing is an excerpt from a broader description, but it represents an attempt to provide a sample of what "knowing about what's going on here" in the form of descriptions of lived experience has to offer nurses. Understanding and interventions in patient support, teaching, and planning for the "unplanned" when we encounter parents who may be bearing children in later years needs to be founded on the answer to the question, What's it like for couples who have delayed pregnancy? In a larger context, our interventions need to be based on answers to the question, What's it like to be pregnant at different phases in the life cycle? The humanistic themes of context and individuality become apparent when we articulate clearly that differences may exist in the lived experience of pregnancy according to when pregnancy occurs in the life cycle. This may sound fundamental, but qualitative designs for studying specific phenomena like Sauer's, clearly bring to awareness some of the essences and interrelationships of lived experiences.

In Summary

Both Oiler and Sauer have presented nurse researchers with descriptions that reflect the influence of a phenomenological perspective. The descriptions as presented here are, of course, encapsulated; to appreciate the richness and the significance of the contributions, the reader will want to study the primary sources.

Oiler and Sauer explored lived experiences as described by those who experienced them through their articulated perceptions. As we move on now to grounded theory, we will see many of the same philosophical underpinnings permeating this qualitative design, but with an emphasis on formulating concepts and theory.

GROUNDED THEORY

The grounded theory method of research goes beyond describing an event or situation to conceptualizing it. Stern (1980) states that grounded theory "aims to generate theoretical constructs which explain the action in the social context under study" (p. 21). The intent of this method is to develop concepts that are abstractions grounded in the data and set off with specific definitions (Diers, 1979). Glaser and Strauss developed the grounded theory method in the 1960s. These two sociologists, whose works have significantly influenced their own field and many nurse researchers (Benoliel, Hutchinson, Swanson & Chenitz, Stern, Wilson), have provided the method to go about formulating theories at the first level of theory development. Examples of their work include *Awareness of Dying* (1965) and *Time for Dying* (1967), as well as in a book on the method itself, *Discovery of Grounded Theory* (1967).

Like phenomenology, the grounded theory method is most useful when little is known about a topic and few theories, if any, exist to explain a phenomenon. Hutchinson (1986), in a description of grounded theory, states:

> Grounded theory utilizes an inductive, from the ground-up approach using everyday behaviors or organizational patterns to generate theory. Such a theory is inherently relevant to the world from which it emerges, whereas the relevance of verification research (second level inquiry) varies widely. (p. 113)

Norris (1982), who also uses the terms "comparative analysis" and "idea testing" for grounded theory methodology, says that this design

> proves useful not only for the discovery of substantive theory but also for the clarification of theoretical building blocks, or nursing concepts. (p. 41).

Stern (1985) places this design within context:

> Nurse scientists who use grounded theory find it ideal for teaching nursing problems. . . . Because the scientist generates constructs (or theory) from the data rather than applying a theory constructed by someone else from another data source, the generated theory remains connected to or grounded in the data. (p. 149)

One of the basic assumptions in grounded theory is that there are unidentified concepts or constructs that, if identified, will enable understanding and problem solving. As with the preceding methods, language varies. What we generally refer to as concepts or constructs are referred to in the grounded theory literature as core variables or basic social processes (BSPs). Wilson (1985) states:

> Despite the diversity that characterizes qualitative data, the grounded theory approach presumes the possibility of discovering fundamental patterns in all of social life. (p. 416)

These patterns are called basic social processes, and because they are not as yet articulated, they are not accessible for problem solving or theory development. For example, Hutchinson (1986) identified a basic social process she called "creating meaning" in response to an unarticulated problem that she assumed existed in neonatal intensive care units. The social psychological problem for nurses of dealing with what Hutchinson termed "horror" resulting from dealing repeatedly with deformities and deaths among newborns was solved by the BSP of "creating meaning." This will be discussed further in the description of her study, below. Wilson's study (1982, 1986) identified the BSP of "infracontrolling" to describe how social order is maintained among schizophrenics living under conditions of freedom. She further developed concepts of "presencing," "farring," and "limiting intrusion" to enable the process of developing propositions and theories.

The Grounded Theory Method

Again, it is beyond the intent of this chapter to provide in detail the actual steps of the grounded theory method. Rather, a general idea as to the process is provided and, as with all methods, the reader is referred to additional references and to a "grounded theorist." The steps listed below represent a compilation of Stern's (1985), Wilson's (1985), and Hutchinson's (1986) grounded theory procedures.

(1) *The research problem:* The purpose of the study is to *identify* problems, therefore the researcher does not start with a research problem. The question could be, What are the basic social and psychological processes that explain interaction in a particular setting or under certain conditions?

(2) *Literature search:* This is considered disadvantageous, because it can lead to premature closure of ideas, prejudgments, and an inaccurate aim when participating in the social process.

(3) *Data gathering:* Data collection generally follows the pattern of field research, with the researcher finding him- or herself on the subjects' "home ground." As in ethnographic research, the researcher immerses him- or herself in the social environment. The form this takes varies according to what is necessary and possible, and what fulfills necessary requirements for meaningful interaction. "Bracketing," described in the discussion of phenomenology, is also used in grounded theory, so that "objectivity" in the form of an open mind is possible.

(4) *Data recording:* Whether field notes or recordings are used, the data are eventually coded and categorized as the researcher searches for clarification of the phenomenon and a way to describe it. Coding—applying labels to what is going on—usually utilizes verbs. Stern (1985) gives these examples: "side-stepping, tuning in, tuning out, labelling, selling, teaching" (p. 155). The coded data are compared until patterns and categories emerge. Placing data within categories is a hypothetical pro-

cess, but when performed correctly, it leads to concept development. Coding in words expresses "what is going on" and develops terms to describe dimensions, properties, conditions, strategies, and consequences. Glaser (1978) identifies "families of theoretical codes"; this work is essential reading for a grounded theorist. "Memoing" is a spontaneous activity in which the researcher records his or her ideas in order to capture elusive and shifting connections. A memo in this sense is a recording of a spontaneous thought process, and not a formal, filed note of description.

(5) *Discovering the overriding analytic theme:* Within this process, categories are reduced, sorting takes place so that coherence can generate ideas, and a core category is identified. The researcher searches through the data, codes, and memos for what seems central, what recurs, and what makes sense to the people in the setting. Many researchers diagram a set of interrelationships when writing up their final analysis. (We will see this below for the BSP of "creating meaning.")

(6) *The research report:* The BSP serves as the central focus of the proposed descriptive theory that seeks to describe the basic social processes occurring in a given context. When reworking and writing the theory, the researcher can incorporate relevant literature. Many nurse researchers, when reporting grounded theory, do so by identifying the problem they uncovered within the situation and the BSP that was discovered in operation. Hypotheses can then be generated from these findings. Examples of this include Stern's studies on stepfather families, Pyler and Stern's discovery of "nursing gestalt," Wilson's previously mentioned study, and Benoliel's study on the dying patient.

Glaser/Strauss and Hutchinson

Using Glaser and Strauss's steps from grounded theory method, Hutchinson has conducted many studies. The one briefly described here is titled "Creating Meaning out of Horror" (1984). An outline of the study is presented here.

(1) *Question:* "What is going on in the neonatal intensive care unit?" was the question asked by administrators concerned with NICU nurses' low morale and high turnover rates. Hutchinson agreed to study the situation.

(2) *Method:* Over a period of three months, Hutchinson spent 20 hours a week as a participant observer in a 16-bed NICU.

(3) *Findings:* After implementing the procedures of data collection developed by Glaser and Strauss, Hutchinson found that nurses had to cope with the social psychological problem of facing the stress that comes with caring for newborns with extreme deformities, who were subjected to extreme treatments, and who died. The core variable, or BSP, that she described in her theory was called "creating meaning." When nurses

failed to create meaning in their work, they experienced burnout, depression, and low morale. If they were able to create meaning, nurses obtained a satisfaction that enabled them to continue in the face of what was described as "horror." Implications of this study come from the recognition that finding ways to assist nurses in "creating meaning" would indeed be a worthwhile goal to pursue.

(4) *Diagram of the major theoretical codes for NICU research:* The following diagram illustrates the interrelationships and integration of the concepts. It is a model of the theory.

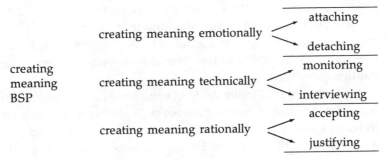

Objectivity, Reliability, and Validity

Objectivity is the essential basis of all good research, including qualitative designs. In the scientific world, however, the assumption seems to exist that we all use the word *objectivity* in the same way, as though it has a fixed universal definition (i.e., the definition associated with positivistic science). Kirk and Miller (1986) offer this contrasting definition:

> Objectivity is the simultaneous realization of as much reliability and validity as possible. Reliability is the degree to which the finding is independent of accidental circumstances of the research, and validity is the degree to which the finding is interpreted in a correct way. (p. 20)

Refocusing our perspective somewhat from the traditional view of objectivity, where the researcher is separate from his or her research or at least not contaminating it, is important in understanding the concepts of objectivity in qualitative designs. Though the researcher is a primary "instrument" in qualitative designs, this presence is aimed at coming as close as possible to a reality or lived experience as it occurs in its natural unfolding. The steps for the two qualitative designs described include measures for acknowledging, dealing with, and lay-ing aside the researcher's values, biases, and preconceptions. They are laid out at the beginning of the study, as part of a good design. The literature review is postponed to further this effort. The researcher makes every effort to clear his or her perceptual field so that he or she can absorb experience as fresh, new, and unbiased. To do this completely, of course, is impossible, but the attempt is aimed at the "realization of as much reliability and validity as possible."

"Instruments" other than humans are also filled with values, biases, preconceptions, and other hindrances to objectivity. More important to theory development in nursing—and to the questions of objectivity, reliability, and validity—is the use of instruments developed in one context or environment to test hypotheses with populations in other cultures or contexts.

With the two qualitative designs presented here, a researcher could have instead chosen from a number of life or work satisfaction scales to reach some conclusion about nurses' experiences, or about having a child later in life. But (and here is my bias) would this produce the richness in data and detail, the authenticity, the "real-life" dimensions that qualitative designs offer us?

The question of reliability and validity remains even when the researcher reports "unbiased" perceptions. We can all view or participate in the same event and each tell the story of what occurred very differently. That is why the steps in a qualitative design ask the researcher to reflect on personal foundations and intuitions. But what about different versions of the same event? Qualitative researchers see this as part of the context, part of the "objective" world. Differing perceptions, for example, about any lived experience play an essential part in any study. What we are seeking is a faithful representation of what is happening, and that, of course, may be different for different individuals; *that* then becomes part of what is happening in a lived experience.

If we dispense with using the word *objectivity* with the meaning that the positivists assign it, our ideas for validity and reliability can be reinterpreted. Currently, the same criteria used to evaluate the scientific method, as we commonly call the positivist view of the world, are used to evaluate qualitative methods that are based on an entirely different worldview (see Brink, 1989). Leininger (1985) presents a good argument for applying different criteria when evaluating the reliability and validity of qualitative research. She contends that *validity* in qualitative research refers to "gaining knowledge and understanding of the true nature, essence, meaning, attributes, and characteristics of a particular phenomenon under study. Measurement is not the goal" (p. 68).

Sampling

With a qualitative design, the sample is considered that part of reality that is observed and recorded. There is a research focus or research question and the researcher proceeds to sample until satisfied that the richness of the data is accurate and meaningful to report. Because there are no statistical requirements mandating a specific number of subjects, the goals of reliability and validity guide the sampling process. A case study with an N of one may provide the seed of an important theory. A sample of one NICU, as in Hutchinson's report discussed above, provides a basis for further comparison and exploration. One guideline that may be helpful (if not always practical) in determining sample size is to continue to collect data within the research focus until no new information is obtained (see Morse, 1989).

HUMAN SUBJECTS ISSUES

Informed consent, type of participation by the researcher, differentiating roles, "off the record" remarks, and "unwelcome results" must be attended to in qualitative methods. Methods textbooks for each qualitative design give suggestions and guidelines for handling these problems. There are special ethical considerations to be taken into account when utilizing qualitative designs (see Munhall, 1988, 1989; Punch, 1986).

CONCLUDING REMARKS

The challenges of qualitative research can be metaphorically likened to the challenges facing any explorer: the unknown, the unforeseen, the unpredictable. The whole idea of discovery involves not knowing what you are about to come upon, unveil, and bring to consciousness. In this chapter, the opportunities to explore phenomena through the qualitative designs of phenomenology and grounded theory are presented to stimulate and guide the reader through uncharted waters.

The aim of this chapter has not been to provide a definitive methods map, but rather to generate enthusiasm and interest in qualitative designs as additional ways of studying nursing phenomena. These designs can enrich our understanding and descriptions of human responses and human experiences in a humanistic scientific dialect. I have found these qualitative designs to be enormously meaningful, lending an authentic type of insight, enriching me and enabling me to know people in ways I never thought possible.

NOTE

1. This section is reprinted from Munhall, P. L. (1989). Philosophical ponderings on qualitative research methods in nursing. *Nursing Science Quarterly*, 2(1), 20-28. Copyright © by William & Wilkins, 1980. Reprinted by permission.

REFERENCES

Benoliel, J. (1967). *The nurse and the dying patient*. New York: Macmillan.
Benoliel, J. (1984). Advancing nursing science: Qualitative approaches. *Western Journal of Nursing Research*, 7(1), 1-8.
Brink, P. (1989). Issues in reliability and validity. In J. Morse (Ed.), *Qualitative nursing research*. Rockville, MD: Aspen.
Chesler, P. (1979). *With child: A diary of motherhood*. New York: Thomas Crowell.
Diers, D. (1979). *Research in nursing practice*. Philadelphia: J. B. Lippincott.
Field, P., & Morse, J. (1985). *Nursing research: The application of qualitative approaches*. Rockville, MD: Aspen.
Glaser, B., & Strauss, A. (1965). *Awareness of dying*. Chicago: Aldine.
Glaser, B., & Strauss, A. (1967). *The discovery of grounded theory*. Chicago: Aldine.
Glaser, B., & Strauss, A. (1968). *Time for dying*. Chciago: Aldine.
Hutchinson, S. (1984). Creating meaning out of horror. *Nursing Outlook*, 32(2), 86-90.
Hutchinson, S. (1985). Perspective: Field research in a neonatal intensive care unit. *Topics in Clinical Nursing*, 7(2), 24-28.
Hutchinson, S. (1986). Grounded theory: The method. In P. Munhall & C. Oiler (Eds.), *Nursing research: A qualitative perspective*. (pp. 111-129). Norwalk, CT: Appleton-Century-Crofts.
Kirk, J., & Miller, M. L. (1986). *Reliability and validity in qualitative research*. Beverly Hills, CA: Sage.
Leininger, M. (Ed.). (1985). *Qualitative research methods in nursing*. New York: Grune & Stratton.
Morse, J. (Ed.). (1989). *Qualitative nursing research: A contemporary dialogue*. Rockville, MD: Aspen.

Munhall, P. (1988). Ethical considerations in qualitative research. *Western Journal of Nursing Research, 10*(2), 150-162.

Munhall, P. (1989a). Institutional review: A task of no small consequence. In J. Morse (Ed.), *Qualitative nursing research: A contemporary dialogue.* Rockville, MD: Aspen.

Munhall, P. (1989b). Philosophical ponderings on qualitative research methods in nursing. *Nursing Science Quarterly, 2*(1), 20-28.

Munhall, P., & Oiler, C. (Eds.). (1986). *Nursing research: A qualitative perspective.* Norwalk, CT: Appleton-Century-Crofts.

Norris, C. (1982). *Concept clarification in nursing.* Rockville, MD: Aspen.

Oiler, C. (1982). The phenomenological approach in nursing research. *Nursing Research, 31*, 118-131.

Oiler, C. (1983). Nursing reality as reflected in nurses' poetry. *Perspectives in Psychiatric Care, 21*, 81-89.

Omery, A. (1983). Phenomenology: A method for nursing research. *Advances in Nursing Science, 5*(2), 49-63.

Parse, R., Coyne, A., & Smith, M. J. (1985). *Nursing research: Qualitative methods.* Bowie, MD: Brady.

Punch, M. (1986). *The politics and ethics of fieldwork.* Beverly Hills, CA: Sage.

Reinharz, S. (1983). Phenomenology as a dynamic process. *Phenomenology and Pedagogy, 1*, 77-79.

Sauer, J. (1985). Using a phenomenological method to study nursing phenomena. In M. Leininger (Ed.), *Qualitative research methods in nursing* (pp. 93-107). New York: Grune & Stratton.

Spiegelberg, W. (1976). *The phenomenological movement* (2 vols.). The Hague: Martinus Nijhoff.

Stern, P. (1980). Grounded theory methodology: Its use and processes. *Image, 12*, 20-23.

Stern, P. (1985). Using grounded theory method in nursing research. In M. Leininger (Ed.), *Qualitative research methods in nursing* (pp. 149-160). New York: Grune & Stratton.

Swanson, J. M., & Chenitz, W. C. (1986). *From practice to grounded theory: Qualitative research.* Menlo Park, CA: Addison-Wesley.

Wilson, H. S. (1982). *Deinstitutionalized residential approaches for the severely mentally disordered patient: The Soteria House approach.* New York: Grune & Stratton.

Wilson, H. S. (1985). *Research in nursing.* Menlo Park, CA: Addison-Wesley.

Wilson, H. S. (1986). Presencing: Doing grounded theory. In P. Munhall & C. Oiler (Eds.), *Nursing research: A qualitative perspective* (pp. 131-144). Norwalk, CT: Appleton-Century-Crofts.

Zbilut, J. P. (1977). Linguistic constraints in nursing practice. *Forum, 16*, 339-342.

PART V

OTHER TYPES OF DESIGNS

This section is devoted to designs that either cross-cut our paradigm or deserve special attention of their own. Historical designs could have been discussed as descriptive designs that use content analysis of available data, but historiography has been used by historians exclusively for a long time. Our definition of descriptive studies has its antecedents in the social sciences rather than the humanities, so we felt it best to give the historical method its own chapter, authored by Laurie Glass.

We have long been intrigued with the idea that epidemiologic methods and procedures are natural and appropriate for nursing research. For this reason we have given special attention to this design by giving it a chapter of its own, written by Janet Meininger.

Evaluation research has become necessary for many health care agencies as quality assurance in health care has become a critical issue. Hospital accreditation boards, licensing agencies, and stockholders all want to know whether the objectives of the institution are being met and to what degree. There are references available on this research approach that are usable for nursing settings, and so we offer a review of the literature on evaluative design in the chapter by Marilynn Wood.

Almost every researcher, at one time or another, has felt frustrated by the lack of instrumentation available for specific study purposes and has, as a result, designed a new instrument. Most of these data collection devices have little more than face validity and are tested for reliability within the context of the study itself, if at all, giving little credence to the findings and often ruining an otherwise good study (Osguthorpe, Roper, & Saunders, 1983; Risser, Strong, & Bither, 1980). For this reason, the chapter on methodological research has been provided by Merle Mishel to demonstrate how to develop research instruments that

181

are both reliable and valid. Methodological research is serious business, not a hit-or-miss affair.

Finally, we include a brief chapter on the pilot study by Nancy Lackey and Anita Wingate, as this is a neglected subject in most research texts. Although authors have consistently placed pilot studies under the exploratory design heading, we feel the pilot study is not limited to the exploratory level. Indeed, if a pilot or feasibility study is not planned for all levels of research, the final study is likely to be flawed. We heard this paper presented at the 1987 Midwest Nursing Research Society meeting and liked it. We hope you do too.

REFERENCES

Osguthorpe, N., Roper, J., & Saunders, J. (1983). The effect of teaching on medication knowledge. *Western Journal of Nursing Research, 5*(3), 205-216.

Risser, N. L., Strong, A., & Bither, S. (1980). Postoperative ventilatory function: A self critique. *Western Journal of Nursing Research, 2*(2), 484-500.

9. Historical Research

Laurie K. Glass

The historical method of research is the process of critically examining and analyzing records of the past. Historiography is the imaginative reconstruction of the past from the data derived by this process. Although historical research is a respected method of inquiry, it has not always been popular in nursing. However, there has been a resurgence of interest in this area in the past few years.

According to Notter (1972), ''Historical research is not merely a collection of incidents, facts, dates, or figures; it is a study of the relationships of facts and incidents, of themes or currents of social and professional issues that have influenced past events and continue to influence the present and future'' (p. 483). Specifically, historical research is conducted for one of the following reasons: to discover the unknown; to answer the question, Why?; to look for implications or relationships to the present; and to communicate the past accomplishments of individuals as well as the profession. This last reason to study history serves the secondary purpose of instilling pride and esprit de corps in the members of the profession.

One basic assumption underlying the use of this method is that the study of the past is valuable and provides useful information for the present. Without a belief in retrospective analysis it is difficult to justify the use of the historical method. An additional assumption is that data are available. Unlike other methods, historical research relies strictly on data created by someone other than the researcher. If records (data) have not been generated and retained, no information exists on which to base an investigation. In the historical method the researcher acts as the instrument, in that the data are all filtered through the investigator before being identified as significant or insignificant. The strength of the results hinges on the belief that a researcher will be guided by the research questions and maintain an objective view of the data. While plowing through mountains of data, the researcher must remain conscious of the need to retrieve all relevant data and not just the data that answer research questions to the researcher's liking. Historical research should be a clear, unbiased quest for answers.

THE BASIC DESIGN

The basic method for historical analysis involves locating and examining documents, interpreting the evidence, and explaining the response. Seven steps are identifiable:

(1) Think about and define a question.
(2) Identify the secondary sources.
(3) Locate and read the secondary sources.
(4) Frame and focus the research questions.
(5) Identify and locate the primary sources.
(6) Utilize the primary sources.
(7) Conduct analysis, synthesis, and exposition.

The initial question is usually broad. It may reflect an area of interest, for example, Why did this school give so many different kinds of degrees? Or, Who was Laura Logan? The investigator then needs to identify the secondary sources, which implies finding what has been written on the area of interest. Secondary sources include books, monographs, articles, and similar items written about the subject. With historical topics, this often means paging through journals of the era looking for news items, or examining history books about institutions and organizations with which an individual or issue was associated. The investigator reads as much as can be found on the subject and related organizations, events, and people. As the investigator learns more about the subject, he or she can identify specific questions to be answered.

The questions so formulated are specifically focused and provide a framework for the research. The breadth and depth of the project will determine the number of questions to be answered. These questions also guide the researcher in examining the primary sources since data are sought from these sources to answer the questions.

Identifying primary sources involves discovering and locating manuscript collections that include pertinent historical documents. Primary sources are those that contain the words of a witness to or first recorder of an event. Examples include minutes, diaries, correspondence, manuscripts, and speeches. Primary sources can be located using published indexes to manuscript collections, or by communicating with agencies and organizations about the location of their historical records. Established archival agencies usually have inventories for each collection, which facilitates the location of specific items or files.

Gathering information from primary sources is considered the actual "data collection." Volumes of data are examined in the search for answers to the focused questions. Significant data are recognized by their relationship to or fit with the whole picture, or by repeated findings that identify trends or patterns. Each document is judged using external and internal criticism (validity and reliability). This means that all documents must be judged for authenticity and credibility. Notes are meticulously kept, not only on the content of the document but on the document itself and its location.

During the analysis, synthesis, and exposition phase of the historical research process, the data are interpreted. The researcher reviews the data thoroughly, categorizing it according to topic or theme and then reconstructing the results into a response that answers the questions. Interpretation is based in the time period of the events discussed. Supplementary data on events, organizations, or people that surface during the use of both secondary and primary sources is sought and used to further explain situations. If an argument is proposed, the support or refutation of that argument lies in the strength of the data. The analysis and synthesis of the data are largely intellectual tasks grounded in the researcher's knowledge and experience with the topic. Exposition involves writing the narrative story that results from the interpretation (analysis and synthesis) of the data. Footnotes are utilized to document sources, explain statements, or to provide verification and make possible additional research by an interested reader. The exposition of the research is considered the "art" of history. The report may be written as a story that is pleasant to read yet is based on sound research.

Degree of Control over the Data

In historical research, the degree of control over the data can be discussed both from the vantage point of the creation and existence of the data as well as from that of the use of the data. The investigator has no control over the creation of the data or the environment in which it was created. The data either exist or do not exist. If the information sought was not recorded and saved, then there are no data. It is possible for some historical research questions to go unanswered because data do not exist. The saving and storage of the data also lie outside the control of the investigator. Documents may be discarded as useless, or may be stored in conditions that hasten their deterioration. The investigator is thus dependent upon the actions of others for the data.

In order to use the data, the investigator must travel to the data. The data are under the control of the agency where they are stored. For nursing history, this may be an archive, historical society, or hospital. The investigator has access to the data only under the conditions defined by the controlling agency. Brooks's (1969) review of the most common regulations and rules concerning historical data should be required reading for every neophyte historical researcher. The most overriding condition is that most of these agencies are open, and thus the data are available, Monday through Friday, 8:00 a.m. to 4:30 p.m. If the investigator must travel some distance to the data and the amount of time that can be spent with the data is limited, the pursuit of the research can become expensive, in both time and money. At this pont the data almost control the investigator, because data access is controlled by the owners of the data. The investigator must work within the structure provided by the agency housing the data and must alter his or her schedule and design the work to ensure the most efficient quest for data.

While using the data, the researcher does have control over the process of defining what constitutes significant information. As records and manuscripts are perused, information most significant to the problem at hand is retrieved. As information is selected from the volumes of documents examined, these items become the data that will be used for the analysis and synthesis. The investigator has complete control here by defining what is important and selecting from the records what he or she deems significant. As mounds of notes are carried away, the situation becomes one in which the investigator has complete control over the data and their interpretation.

To summarize, the investigator has no control over the creation and storage of the documents that become data. However, he or she has total control over the selection of what information in the documents will become data for the research project.

NURSING PROBLEMS SUITED TO HISTORICAL METHODS

The historical method has been used in nursing research to reconstruct events, to analyze the rationale behind decisions, to trace activities and influences leading to current events, to analyze the scientific base and origin of procedures, to discover the impetus and sequencing of events, to analyze a person's ideas, to interpret the influence of a leader, and to understand nursing within the realm of the social, economic, political, and cultural setting of the time. Although many readers may think of history as a chronology of dates and places, historical research relies heavily on the analytical and interpretive skill of the investigator.

In their research on the experience of nurses as prisoners of war, Kalisch and Kalisch (1976) not only reconstructed a series of events, they placed them within the setting and cultural scene that existed at the time. By describing the situation that existed before the occurrence of the main event (nurses taken prisoner), they provide the reader with a sense of the "normal" situation and introduce the key factors in that situation. Using a chronological framework, they then describe and interpret the events that subsequently occurred, and the reactions of the nurses. For data, they relied upon newspaper and journal articles by nurses and correspondents at the scene, books (primarily diaries and biographies) published after the war, and government reports. The writing style of their report gives the reader a sense of being in the situation with those unfortunate nurses. In the end, Kalisch and Kalisch accomplish their task of discovering what the experience was and reconstructing it so that others might learn from it. Knowledge has been gained in the areas of military nursing, ingenuity and creativity in times of stress, the needs of wartime nursing, and World War II.

My own work on Katharine Densford Dreves illustrates the importance of studying the people who have contributed to the nursing profession (Glass, 1984). As a nursing leader, Dreves's (1890-1978) professional life spans a time of great importance for nursing. The original purpose of the research was to discover who Katharine Densford Dreves was and what her influence had been on the profession. The final analysis yielded relevant data on professional organizations, nursing research in the 1930s, the profession's response to the need for nurses during World War II, and an individual's professional commitment. The basic data for the research were located in the Katharine Densford Dreves Papers at the University of Minnesota Archives. Available sources included diaries, extensive private and professional correspondence, speeches, manuscripts, and photographs. These data were supplemented with additional primary data from institutional and organizational records (such as the university president's papers and the School of Medicine's records). Secondary sources (books, journal articles) provided additional information related to the events and concerns of the era. This project required three years of source utilization and analysis. The results not only reconstruct the past but also contribute new knowledge in a number of areas.

During the analysis of Dreves's life from early childhood until her entry into nursing, it was possible to identify factors that contributed to her ability to become a leader. In addition, the analysis of her later life as a nursing leader led to the identification of distinct characteristics of her leadership style. This study has contributed to knowledge of leadership behaviors and women as leaders. An analysis of Dreves's status as an educated single woman during a time when women were expected to be in the home also provides insight into the struggles of someone breaking ground in uncharted territory. A contribution also has been made to documenting the history of women. A large project such as this can be partitioned into smaller topics to ensure a more in-depth analysis or to stimulate additional related research.

Dreves's work on a specific project over a four-year time span is discussed in "Raising a Million Dollars: Katharine Densford Dreves and the American Nurses Foundation" (Glass, 1985). This particular episode in history could be analyzed and recounted in a paper of reasonable length, unlike larger projects that require years of study and volumes to communicate. Located in the Dreves Papers was extensive correspondence with the American Nurses Foundation staff, state nurses' association members, foundation donors, and national nursing leaders. Dreves also kept brochures, press releases, financial reports, and internal organizational memos and reports. These items provided a wealth of information about the Foundation and the roles played by Dreves and her husband. The archived records of the American Nurses Foundation (at the Nursing Archives, Boston University) contained little new information. Major activities also could be verified through nursing journals. In total, there was a stack of 10-12 inches of usable material (about 2,000 pieces of paper). From this material it was possible to reconstruct the fund-raising campaign, identify the key players, ascertain Dreves's motivation and commitment to the campaign, and identify an emerging concern with nursing research. The significance of Dreves's work with the Foundation is emphasized by the reputation and activities of the Foundation today and by the fact that this was the first fund-raising campaign conducted for the American Nurses Foundation. The report of this project not only provides previously unknown information, but also describes fund-raising methods that could be used today.

STRENGTHS AND WEAKNESSES OF THE METHOD

The historical method can be used to answer questions and to contribute to the solution of nursing problems. However, it rarely stops with nursing concerns, because the content dealt with must be considered within the context in which it occurred. Nursing's concerns do not occur in a vacuum, but within societal, political, and economic arenas. Using the historical method to answer nursing questions also facilitates answering questions in other areas, such as women's activities, education, role development, and institutional development. The strength of the method lies in its applicability to diverse topics and the breadth of knowledge that can be discovered through its use.

The historical method relies on the critical examination and analysis of materials. The individual investigator is the sole finder and analyzer of the data. The analysis is dependent upon the intellectual processes used by the investigator. In order to conduct a study, the investigator assumes there are adequate data to answer the question. The sources of data are classified, organized, and stored according to a system developed by an archivist. There is a certain amount of inflexibility to the data, as they may not be in the form that the investigator wants. Since they were created b someone else, the data exist in a form that was useful to the originator and not necessarily to the investigator. For example, the data may be in the form of annual statistics when the researcher desires monthly statistics, or the data might be located in committee minutes that are labeled and stored in an unusual manner.

Access to data also can be an item of concern. Archival data are located in public and private agencies. Each sector has rules regarding access to and use of the records for research. Access is more difficult to achieve in private agencies such as hospitals, visiting nurse associations, or professional associations because usage is controlled by the current executive officer unless policies have been established. The investigator might have to seek permission from the original donor or the chief administrator to review the documents. After the materials have been located and access assured, the researcher needs to be concerned with policies concerning how the records may be used and the information retained. Variations on usage rules include allowing reading only, reading and note taking, and photocopying.

The historical method can be expensive and time-consuming. Since the investigator must travel to the data, transportation and lodging expenses can become a burden if the data are located in numerous cities. The researcher must also have blocks of time available in which to travel and review the data. When traveling to the data, the researcher must allow enough time to account for finding more data than was anticipated, so that additional trips may be avoided.

Reviewing thousands of pieces of paper to determine the significance of the content is a time-consuming task. Because so much of the location and analysis of data is an intellectual process implemented by the investigator, it is not feasible to hire research assistants to help with the project during this phase.

Given sufficient time, funding, and data, the historical method can be an exciting and satisfying process for the nursing investigator. However, because records often are stored in out-of-the-way places and archives are often located in basements, pursuit of historical research is not for those with allergies to dust, dirt, or mold.

MODEL

The historical method is used primarily for descriptive studies and theory building. An inductive approach to data collection is used. In the case of theory building, the investigator presents an interpretation for confirmation or argument and criticism. The best examples of theory building in nursing history are those arguments presented by Ashley (1976) and Melosh (1982). Each investigator presents data and an interpretation of how the nursing profession has developed as a work force. Ashley (1976) concluded that nursing's development was limited by oppressive and paternalistic environmental forces (primarily physician-dominated hospitals). Melosh (1982) suggests that nursing's development was affected by a split between the nursing leaders and working nurse. The conclusions of these authors are interestingly different and invite criticism.

SAMPLES

Samples and sampling techniques as traditionally defined are not commonly used in historical research. If an investigator discovers a massive data set in an archival setting and determines that it is not necessary to analyze the entire field of data, he or she may choose to sample the data set. For example, if 2,000 wills are available, the investigator might choose every fifth will for content analysis. An investigator also might determine a unit of analysis if the data for the project are plentiful and cut across settings or groups. For example, an investigator may choose to review the nursing committee minutes for January 1945 for each hospital in Chicago to analyze working nurses' responses to a possible draft of nurses. In this instance, the unit of analysis would be each set of nursing committee minutes.

These examples represent rare occurrences in historical research. The investigator's concern is to locate sufficient primary data to answer the research questions. To do this, times, places, events, and people related to the research questions are identified. Indexes to manuscript collections and telephone calls or letters to organizations and people can be used to discover the actual physical location of relevant sources. In addition, journal indexes and books published near the time of interest might provide clues to sources of data. The research questions determine the quest for data. If the questions are specific to a person, place, or thing, the search for data sources may not be as extensive as for broad, general questions. In the study of an individual's life, data sources may be compact, or they may be spread about widely. The papers of Katharine Densford Dreves were located in one place because she was primarily associated with one institution. The papers of Laura

Logan are located in seven different places because she tended to change jobs. Research may involve utilizing all locatable data, or collecting as many data as needed to answer the question. When the same information is found repeatedly in the data, the quest for additional data ceases.

METHODS OF DATA COLLECTION

The main method of data collection in historical research is the critical examination of documents. However, the investigator might also interview relevant people, review and analyze videotapes or films, visit sites of events, and examine artifacts.

Issues with Secondary Document Sources

Secondary sources are documents written by others about the research question or a related area. Items included in this category are books, journal articles, newspaper articles (including obituary notices), and films. To identify these sources, the researcher uses cumulative indexes to the published literature, reference lists in historically significant books, and computerized search programs such as HISLINE (National Library of Medicine medical history resource citations). Since the major cumulative indexes for nursing literature begin with the 1950s, a hand search through the pages of the journals published prior to this time may be the only reasonable way to locate pertinent articles. To do a thorough job of this, the investigator must be familiar with the journals published during the years of interest and must know the words used to describe the phenomena at that time. Language changes over time, as does the popularity of words, and both retrieval and recognition (during hand searches) are affected by language familiarity. Making a list of terms in bold print and keeping it visible during the search facilitates the recognition of significant items.

In order to review the secondary sources, the researcher may have to rely on interlibrary loan services, since older books and journals are not readily available in some libraries. Historical societies and used book stores are also excellent resources for the location of old materials. Under the right circumstances (depending upon availability and price) it is sometimes easier to buy a resource than to borrow it, since restraints are often placed on the usage of old materials that are valued.

Changing technology creates a special issue when the investigator is using films and audio recordings as data. Unless the film or audio recording is located in an organized archival setting, the equipment needed to view the film or listen to the recording may no longer be available. As technology changes, the ability to retrieve information that was collected with that technology changes. An excellent example of this is the 1935 recording of M. Adelaide Nutting and Florence Nightingale. Victrolas and record players that can play this record are now almost nonexistent. In one institution, the recording was transferred to cassette tape, so that it was usable. This was possible only because an Educational Communications Department employee searched until he discovered an old machine that could play the record.

Issues with Primary Document Sources

The issues related to primary sources include finding the sources, accessing the sources, and judging the sources. Primary sources can be identified and located through the use of indexes, such as the Library of Congress's *National Union Catalog of Manuscript Collections* (NUCMC) or Hinding's (1980) *Women's History Sources: A Guide to Archives and Manuscript Collections in the United States*. Local or state guides also may be available. It might even be necessary to write to institutions that have a specific relationship to the research questions to inquire about records in their possession or about their knowledge of the location of such records.

Once the records have been located, basic questions must be asked before the investigator travels to the site of the data. Is permission needed to review the records? If so, from whom? Is there a special form to be used in requesting permission? How are records organized? Have the records been processed? This is particularly important because the degree of organization of the records directly affects the amount of time the investigator will need to plan on spending looking at the records. Is there an inventory of the collection? This file-by-file listing of the collection is an invaluable tool for locating specific material or at least providing direction for the hunt. Is someone else currently using the data? If someone else is using the collection, the researchers might want to discuss their mutual interests, possible duplication of efforts, or a team approach to their search for specific answers.

During the search for and use of primary sources, the investigator's best friend and ally is the archivist. These people who work professionally to collect, organize, and make accessible the records that provide us with a view of history can provide priceless assistance. Archivists know their collections and can suggest other collections where additional information might be found. If the research questions involve a local problem or person, archivists know their local history and can provide information about people and organizations. Their experience with the organization of records and files also can facilitate problem solving when the researcher is trying to figure out where a certain piece of information might be located. The investigator will benefit from knowing the archivist and talking to the archivist about the research. As professionals, archivists adhere to a code of confidentiality for each researcher's work, so "trade secrets" are never discussed. However, they will refer one investigator to another if there is a crossover in the area of interest. Archivists want their collections to be used (it justifies the storage of all that paper), and generally will go out of their way to be of assistance.

During the actual data collection, the issues are twofold: Are these really usable data? Are these data significant? Each piece of possible evidence is analyzed. To make a decision about the data really being usable, the researcher must judge a document's authenticity and credibility. This is accomplished through external and internal criticism. External criticism questions the authenticity of the document. In other words, is this document really what it appears to be? This judgment is made based on where the document is found and on the handwriting, ink, type, or paper used. The scandal over the so-called Hitler diaries is an example of documents that failed to pass tests of external criticism.

Internal criticism questions the accuracy, meaning, and credibility of the content of the document. Is what it says really what happened? To establish credibility of a document, the investigator must find corroborating evidence to support what is said, for instance, by finding another account of an incident described and comparing the stories.

Recognizing data as significant requires in-depth familiarity with the topic and an alertness when going through the data that is strengthened by practice. Significance is determined by the fit of the data with the whole picture. However, if the data are spread out, the investigator may not initially recognize their significance. For example, in the Dreves Papers what appeared to be the publication of a rather routine nursing textbook on ethics later resurfaced as the source of great controversy. Detailed notes on the location of data facilitate the researcher's return to significant sources when this happens.

Historical researchers also develop a sense of their content when they are immersed in the data for long periods. This sense provides recognition of missing pieces, something that doesn't look quite right, or something that appears to be missing. With the zeal of a detective, the researcher pursues whatever is necessary to get the complete story.

Another clue to significance in data collection is the repetitious citing of a particular idea, act, or event. Repetition can be a sign that a trend or pattern is developing, that an individual's values are reflected in his or her behavior, or that the issue was of concern to a wide audience. The researcher needs to investigate the meaning behind the repetition.

When using primary sources, the researcher may encounter additional problems related to the fact that the data were created by other people. Missing data may mean that records were destroyed and that the data are not retrievable. The filing system and language may be something the investigator has never seen before. Files that may contain relevant and significant information may be restricted in usage or may be sealed until a date 20 years into the future. This is common practice when the records contain information about people who are still alive, or when the records contain information judged to be damaging if released at this time.

Artifacts and Site Visits

A researcher may also find it helpful to examine nontextual items related to the topic. For example, photographs, certificates, medallions, clothing, and equipment can provide a sense of history and reveal interesting bits of information. A visit to the site of a home, meeting, grave, battle, or other event also can enhance the spirit with which an investigator writes about a topic. Because the names of towns and streets change, the researcher should check old city directories for correct locations. When the researcher visits a cemetery, the manager can provide specific information about the location of a grave and the family history at the time of the death.

DATA ANALYSIS

During data collection, the researcher analyzes each possible piece of evidence in order to determine if the document and information it contains is truly solid. This data analysis is different from, yet related to, the analysis that occurs after the primary data have been collected. The actual data analysis occurs through a process of synthesis. According to Austin (1958), "This process involves several problems, such as organization of the data according to some plan, their adequate documentation, the determination of the meaning of the facts, and the discovery of relationships among them—a creative process" (p. 9). The data are sorted into categories and examined for themes, trends, and patterns. The data are interpreted within the time and standards of the era in which they were created. That era may be compared to other eras, but the basic interpretation must be consistent with the time in which the data were generated. This becomes particularly important when analyzing data that are sociologically based, especially with topics such as women's roles and family.

The data might be analyzed and interpreted according to a conceptual framework or the framework formed by the research questions. Support is sought for the premise that led the investigation. It is through the analysis that the groundwork is laid for the argument presented. Unlike other methods, the analysis does not appear on paper. It is a process that goes on in the head of the researcher, who eventually puts ideas on paper in the form of a report. The visual aspect of the data analysis process jumps from the pile of notes to the story. As with a jigsaw puzzle, the pieces are assembled into a picture in order to communicate results.

The mechanics of historical research dictate that data analysis occur at the same time as the exposition, or writing of the report. Reports are narrative and make extensive use of footnotes. Footnotes are essential with this method. They are utilized to explain statements, to acknowledge cited sources, and to document the location of data. Because historians do not have the raw data in their possession and the "experiment" cannot be replicated, footnotes are the key to the verification of the research and the stimuli for additional investigations. Historical reports without footnotes are suspect because a reader cannot determine the validity of the data on which the interpretation was based.

RELIABILITY AND VALIDITY

Reliability and validity issues are pertinent to data collection and interpretation (analysis). The internal and external criticism of the documents during data collection represent an attempt to secure reliable and valid data. External criticism determines the validity or authenticity of the document. It answers the where, when, why, and by whom questions (Christy, 1975). Validity of the document must be ascertained before the reliability of the information contained in it is assessed. Internal criticism questions the reliability of the information contained in the document. Does the researcher understand what is being said? Is what is being said an accurate portrayal of what happened? It is here that the researcher must be alert to possible misinterpretation—either by him- or herself or by the document's author. In his discussion of the principles of historical criticism, Hockett (1955) provides specific ways and means to review for external and internal criticism. External criticism includes determining authorship, finding evidence of dates, detecting spurious documents, and determining the original form. Internal criticism refers to understanding the meaning of the statements and establishing their dependability.

Reliability and validity issues in the data analysis refer to the interpretation made or the argument proposed. The reliability of an interpretation is based on the type of evidence that was found and whether there is enough evidence to support the interpretation. Were the data competently analyzed? Was the researcher aware of possible bias during the analysis? Is the interpretation as objective as it can be? Validity is harder to ascertain. It asks the question, How good an answer is this? The overall aim of historical research is to discover and understand a subject. Reliability and validity questions are related only to the internal consistency and goodness of fit within a study. Comparison between studies is not appropriate unless exactly the same question is being asked.

HUMAN SUBJECTS ISSUES

Historical research occurs primarily through document review. The use of human subjects in the usual sense of a committee review is not an issue unless interviews are scheduled as part of the data collection. There are two related issues particularly relevant to historical research and the involvement of other people.

The first issue revolves around who owns the documents that need to be used. If an archive, library, or business owns the documents that describe an event, this is not an issue. However, if the documents belong to a family and describe activities of family members, then permission is needed to use the documents and the report might be requested for review by the family. This places the researcher in the position of being censored by family members, which is not conducive to scholarly research. The same type of situation might occur when a researcher is writing the history of an organization or institution.

The second issue is the use of information about people who are still alive or who do not know that their names can be found in someone else's archives. This issue is important in the use of papers that contain personal correspondence. If the person mentioned is still alive, the researcher should use professional judgment in detailing the specifics of a topic or disclosing information that may embarrass that individual. If there is any doubt as to whether or not disclosure is an issue, it is best to be conservative; if the information is not crucial to the topic, it should be omitted.

It can come as quite a shock to some individuals that their names exist in archived documents. If a long-standing correspondence between two people is archived without the knowledge of one correspondent, the researcher must use caution in quoting that individual. A basic decision rule for these issues is as follows: If the evidence is truly necessary for the research, the researcher should take the time to find out if the individual is alive and should review the literary property rights laws (Brooks, 1969).

PROPOSAL FEATURES

The key features to be attended to in reviewing proposals for historical research are problem identification, the available sources, and the investigator's qualifications. The problem identified for the research should be delineated in the research questions. It should be specific enough to be answered and to provide a guide, but general enough to be of significance to a broad audience. The problem should be limited in scope to fit within the time line of the investigation. Historical research is more time-consuming than it appears. The background and rationale for investigating the problem should also be stated. The investigator should report everything known about the topic and why the research should occur.

The proposal should indicate that relevant secondary sources have been read and integrated into the background information on the research topic. The proposal also should describe the location, amount, and type of primary sources available to answer the research question. Section headings for a proposal might include the following: Introduction and Background, Purpose, Research Questions, Parameters, Sources, Justification, Time Line, and References.

The investigator should be an experienced historical researcher. Because the historical research design is grounded in the review, analysis, and interpretation of documents by one person, it is important that the investigator be reputable. Formal education and research experience in the historical method establish credibility.

CRITIQUING A REPORT

In critiquing a published research report, the following points should be addressed:[1]

(1) Do the research questions provide a guide or framework for the research? The questions should be specific enough for the reader to understand where the researcher is coming from and where the researcher will go.

(2) What sources did the researcher use? Were sufficient primary sources available for the research? Have secondary sources been used to validate and substantiate the primary sources? The majority of the research should be based on primary sources. Is sufficient documentation presented in the footnotes to allow verification or an attempt at replication?

(3) Are the facts reported satisfactorily to give an honest and clear message? Is the researcher's argument convincing? Is the evidence clearly and logically presented and related to other variables?

(4) Does the writing style make the reader want to continue reading? Is it a smooth style that provides the reader with an enjoyable experience? Are any photographs, tables, or figures used appropriate?

(5) Does the author have the credentials of a historical scholar? Does he or she provide evidence of educational qualifications and other studies?

Historical research reports require the use of the Turabian (1973) style of presentation or that laid out in the University of Chicago's (1982) *Manual of Style*. These styles allow for the inclusion of footnotes and the citation of unpublished sources, a necessity for this method.

Overall, the historical method can be used to explore many topics and to answer many research questions. In nursing, there are ample questions and sufficient primary resources to enable scholarly historical research. The method can be combined with other methods or it can stand alone. It provides an intellectual challenge for the researcher who doesn't mind dust, who likes old things, and who has the skills of an amateur detective.

NOTE

1. I would like to acknowledge as sources for this list the unpublished criteria for evaluating historical research by Janie Brown Novak (1984) and editorial review criteria by Eleanor Pajunen (1985).

REFERENCES

Ashley, J. A. (1976). *Hospitals, paternalism and the role of the nurse.* New York: Teachers College Press.

Austin, A. L. (1958). The historical method in nursing. *Nursing Research, 7,* 4-10.

Barritt, E. R. (1981). Critique: Historical study. In S. D. Krampitz & N. Pavlovich (Eds.), *Readings in nursing research* (pp. 161-163). St. Louis: C. V. Mosby.

Barzun, J., & Graff, H. F. (1985). *The modern researcher* (4th ed.). San Diego, CA: Harcourt Brace Jovanovich.

Brooks, P. C. (1969). *Research in archives: The use of unpublished sources.* Chicago: University of Chicago Press.

Christy, T. E. (1975). The methodology of historical research. *Nursing Research, 24,* 189-192.

Glass, L. K. (1984). Katharine Densford Dreves: Marching at the head of the parade (Doctoral dissertation). *Dissertation Abstracts International, 44,* 3358B.

Glass, L. K. (1985). Raising a million dollars: Katharine Densford Dreves and the American Nurses Foundation. *Journal of Nursing History, 1,* 56-67.

Hinding, A. (Ed.). (1980). *Women's history sources: A guide to archives and manuscript collections in the United States.* Ann Arbor, MI: R. W. Bowker.

Hockett, H. C. (1955). *The critical method in historical research and writing.* Westport, CT: Greenwood.

Kalisch, P. A., & Kalisch, B. J. (1976). Nurses under fire: World War II experiences of nurses on Bataan and Corregidor. *Nursing Research, 25,* 409-425.

Krampitz, S. D. (1981). Research design: Historical. In S. D. Krampitz & N. Pavlovich (Eds.), *Readings in nursing research* (pp. 54-58). St. Louis: C. V. Mosby.

Library of Congress, Descriptive Cataloging Division. (1959-1983). *National union catalog of manuscript collections.* Washington, DC: Author.

Melosh, B. (1982). *The physician's hand: Work culture and conflict in American nursing.* Philadelphia: Temple University Press.

Notter, L. (1972). The case for historical research in nursing. *Nursing Research, 21,* 483.

Turabian, K. L. (1973). *A manual for writers* (4th ed.). Chicago: University of Chicago Press.

University of Chicago Press. (1982). *A manual of style* (13th ed.). Chicago: Author.

10. Epidemiologic Designs

Janet C. Meininger

What is epidemiology? The literal definition of epidemiology is very broad: the study of (logos) what comes upon (epi) the people (demos). It can be defined as the study of the distribution and determinants of health and disease in human population groups.

One of the distinguishing features of epidemiology is that the outcome of interest, the dependent variable, is health or disease status. As the interests of epidemiologists have expanded to include chronic as well as infectious diseases and health as well as disease, models used to explain the incidence of diseases have become more complex. Although the environment has always been an important component in epidemiologic investigations, we now understand that lifestyle factors and the social milieu are related to health status and to the prevention, cause, and course of disease.

Another distinguishing feature of epidemiology is that it is population based. Although individuals are usually the units of analysis, they are studied in the effort to understand the dynamics of health and disease in populations. Characteristically, the epidemiologist measures the frequency of cases in relation to the population in which they occur. The contribution that epidemiologists can make to clinical investigations is increasingly appreciated by both epidemiologists and clinicians. Even in a hospital-based study of patients, the relationship between the sample studied and the target population is of prime interest to the epidemiologist.

Epidemiologists use experimental and observational research designs. Epidemiologic methods have been applied in human experiments involving large populations to test the effectiveness of an intervention on a communitywide basis. The large-scale trial of the polio vaccine is a classic example of this approach (Francis et al., 1955). The Multiple Risk Factor Intervention Trial (MRFIT) is a more recent example of an epidemiologic experiment (Multiple Risk Factor Intervention Trial Research Group, 1982). The experimental method, in which the investigator has control over the independent variable and subjects are randomly assigned to concurrent groups, is not always an ethical or feasible approach to studying health outcomes in human populations. For this reason, epidemiologists have developed and adopted rigorous observational approaches in order to control the myriad sources of bias that can invalidate the study of naturally occurring events. In observational studies, subjects are exposed to the independent variable because of self-selection, genetic endowment, or occupational exposures or those due to geographic location, such as naturally occurring fluoride in the water supply. Subjects otherwise similar who have not been exposed are used for comparison. This emphasis on comparison is another distinguishing feature of epidemiology, but it is by no means unique to it. Because experimentation is not always feasible, epidemiologists rely on careful selection and rigorous comparison of groups that are observed concurrently while controlling extraneous sources of variation. They have also developed guidelines for making causal inferences from epidemiologic studies (Hill, 1965, 1971).

Selected observational designs and methods will be the focus of this chapter. Observational designs are divided into those that are longitudinal and those that are cross-sectional. In a cross-sectional study, all the measurements relate to one point in time, in contrast to the longitudinal approach, in which measurements relate to at least two points in time. In this chapter two longitudinal designs will be discussed: cohort and case-comparison (case-control) studies. The emphasis will be placed on cohort studies since they are much more prevalent in the nursing research literature than case-comparison studies (Jacobsen & Meininger, 1985).

THE LOGIC OF COHORT AND CASE-COMPARISON STUDIES

Although the investigator does not manipulate the independent variable, the logic or flow of reasoning in a cohort study is the same as the logic of an experiment. Subjects are measured or categorized on the basis of the independent variable and are followed forward for observation of the dependent variable. In a cohort study, it is established at the outset that all subjects have not already experienced the outcome of interest (dependent variable). Thus the time sequencing of events can be established; that is, it can be demonstrated that the independent variable preceded the occurrence of the dependent variable.

In a case-comparison study, the logic or flow of reasoning is in the opposite direction. Subjects are categorized on the basis of the dependent variable (the outcome of interest). The purpose of the study is to search for factors in the past (independent variables) that may explain the outcome.

RETROSPECTIVE AND PROSPECTIVE APPROACHES

Formerly, it was common to equate cohort studies with the prospective approach and case-comparison studies with the retrospective approach. This is an oversimplification and is incorrect. *Prospective* and *retrospective* are terms that refer to the timing of the occurrence of the study variables in relation to the investigator's place in time.

A case-comparison study is always retrospective. The investigator begins the study after the occurrence of the dependent variable. Cohort studies, on the other hand, can be conducted prospectively or retrospectively or a combination of both approaches can be used. In a retrospective cohort study (also known as a nonconcurrent follow-up study or a historical cohort study) the dependent variable has already occurred at the time the investigator initiates the study. The sequence of events can be reconstructed through records. Specifically, it can be established that individuals free of the outcome of interest were measured and classified on the basis of the independent variables and can be followed forward in time through the records for documentation of the occurrence of the dependent variable.

COHORT STUDIES

Overview

In a cohort study subjects are selected from a population and then examined to exclude those who have the outcome of interest. In other words, only those at risk of developing the outcome are studied. These individuals are measured and classified in terms of their characteristics (risk factors, exposures, independent variables). The subjects are followed over time to observe the occurrence of the outcome. In the classical epidemiologic study, incidence of disease is the outcome of interest. The analysis consists of comparison of groups with different characteristics (values of the independent variables, risk factors, exposures). The incidence of disease among the exposed is compared with the incidence of disease among the nonexposed. A flowchart for a cohort study is presented in Figure 10.1.

The use of epidemiologic terminology to classify study designs in nursing research is not common. Although the dependent variable is often some aspect of health status, it is not usually a disease entity. Examples of studies that have cohort design features published by nurse researchers include Ballard and McNamara (1983), Jones (1981), Moore (1983), Norbeck and Tilden (1983), and Woods (1980).

Selection of Subjects

Although we usually think of cohorts as birth cohorts—that is, individuals born in a particular year—there are many other kinds of cohorts. Three sources of cohorts are frequently sampled for epidemiologic investigations (MacMahon & Pugh, 1970):

(1) *Special exposure groups* are those receiving especially high doses of a substance hypothesized to have an impact on health outcomes. Examples include occupational groups exposed to chemicals, military groups exposed to herbicides, and survivors of the atomic bomb exposed to radiation.
(2) *Captive subjects* are those who are members of well-defined groups and can be readily contacted and/or followed through records. Examples include members of prepaid health plans, members of professional organizations or other occupational groups, insured persons, obstetric populations receiving prenatal care from a particular source, and students.
(3) *Geographically defined cohorts* are often used in epidemiologic studies. For example, classic studies of cardiovascular disease were based in Framingham, Massachusetts; Evans County, Georgia; and Tecumseh, Michigan.

Those exposed to the independent variable in a cohort study are compared with subjects from the same population who have not been ex-

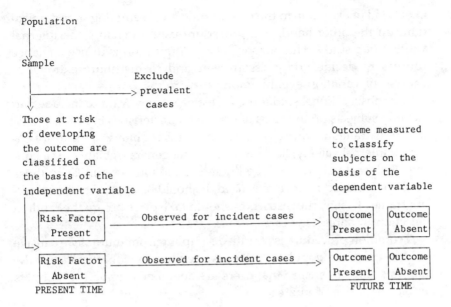

Figure 10.1. Flowchart for a Prospective Cohort Study

posed. Sometimes a comparison group is not readily available. This is the case when an entire group or community has been exposed to something such as an occupational hazard or radiation. In this case, another special cohort is selected on the basis of its being similar to the exposed group. Alternatively, rates for the exposed cohort are compared with rates for the general population. However, even with adjustment for age, sex, and race, comparison of a special cohort with the general population can be invalid because of selection bias.

After an appropriate source of subjects has been decided upon, methods for selecting individuals from these sources are designed. Kelsey, Thompson, and Evans (1986) describe sampling procedures common to epidemiologic studies. The same principles of sample selection apply in this situation as in any other. A random procedure should be used in selection to ensure that each potential subject has the same probability of being selected into the sample. This is not the same as randomization in an experimental study and it does not achieve the same purpose. Random sampling is done to achieve a representative sample in relation to the target population. This is the basis for making statistical inferences about the population from sample data. Application of a statistical test allows the investigator to quantify the likelihood of error due to the chance process of sampling. Randomization, on the other hand, is a procedure used to ensure the internal validity of a study. The purpose of randomization is to use a chance process to decide group assignment and to distribute extraneous sources of variation evenly among the groups.

In an observational study, the investigator may want to include and exclude subjects on the basis of certain characteristics in order to control for extraneous sources of variation. This is done as a means of ensuring internal validity, acknowledging that generalizability of the findings (external validity) will be limited to individuals similar to those studied. If subject restriction is used, it should be applied to the sampling frame. That is, the restriction should take place before the random selection of subjects is carried out.

A common procedure is stratified sampling from mutually exclusive subgroups of the population. This is usually done for efficiency at the analysis stage to ensure that there are adequate numbers of subjects in all categories of interest.

Measures of Effect

The basic structure of the analysis in a cohort study is the comparison of subgroups with different characteristics (independent variables, risk factors, exposures). Comparison of the incidence rates of the outcome in the exposed and unexposed groups is the key feature of the analysis. Table 10.1 displays a 2 × 2 table for dichotomized independent and dependent variables, calculation of the incidence rates for exposed and unexposed groups, and the relative risk, which is one of the measures of effect that can be calculated from cohort data.

The numerator of an incidence rate indicates the number of new cases of the outcome developing over a certain period of time (length of the follow-up period). The denominator in the calculation of an incidence rate indicates the number of individuals at risk of developing the outcome during the follow-up period. Obviously, the denominator does not usually remain stable over the length of the follow-up period, particularly if this period is lengthy. Individuals may drop out, die, or move away, and will no longer be under observation. In addition, individuals may enter the study at slightly different times. For these reasons, the denominator in the calculation of an incidence rate can be expressed as person-time, which takes into account the number of subjects followed and the duration of follow-up for each individual.

Table 10.1   Usual Data Presentation for a Cohort Study

Independent Variable	Dependent Variable		
	Outcome Occurs During Follow-Up Period	Outcome Does Not Occur During Follow-Up Period	Total
Exposed	a	b	a + b
Not exposed	c	d	c + d

$$\text{incidence among those exposed to the independent variable} = \frac{a}{a + b} \times 1000 \text{ per unit time}$$

$$\text{incidence among those not exposed to the independent variable} = \frac{c}{c + d} \times 1000 \text{ per unit time}$$

$$\text{relative risk = ratio of incidence rates} = \frac{\dfrac{a}{a + b}}{\dfrac{c}{c + d}} \text{ per unit time}$$

In a study in which subjects are followed over very long periods of time for the development of chronic diseases with long latency periods such as heart disease and cancer, the denominator is expressed as person-years. In studies with shorter follow-up periods such as investigation of pregnancy outcomes, person-weeks may be the appropriate unit. Person-days is suitable for epidemiologic investigations of acute outbreaks of health problems.

As demonstrated in Table 10.1, relative risk is based on the ratio of incidence rates. Other measures of effect that can be calculated from cohort data are those based on rate differences as opposed to rate ratios. Only the simplest forms of analysis of cohort data are presented to illustrate the structure of an epidemiologic follow-up study and its chief measure of effect, the relative risk. The reader is referred to Elandt-Johnson (1975) for further details on rates and Fleiss (1981), Kelsey et al. (1986), Kleinbaum, Kupper, and Morgenstern (1982), Miettinen (1985), and Rothman (1986) for methods of adjustment for confounding, testing for interaction, analysis of matched data, and subgroup analysis.

Measurement of the Variables

Sources of information about the variables include physical exams; measurements of the environment; self-reports (interviews or responses to standardized tests); clinical, occupational, and school records; and records of births and deaths. As in any other empirical study, the investigator is concerned with the reliability and validity of the measurements. Reliable measures will minimize random errors; valid measures will minimize systematic errors. Methods for assessing reliability and validity depend on the type of instrument used and the level of the resulting measurement. The reader should refer to psychometric texts for background on reliability and validity.

TOWARD AN INTERNALLY VALID STUDY: MINIMIZING BIAS

The design of a study and the methods for carrying it out are aimed at minimizing bias. A study that is sufficiently unbiased is internally valid. Likewise, the research report should include information necessary for a skilled reader to evaluate potential sources of bias and the degree to which internal validity is questionable. It follows that the critique should be targeted toward evaluating these same sources of potential bias.

First, bias will be defined. Three major sources of bias will then be described. Finally, specific examples will be presented to illustrate particular types of bias and steps that can be taken to avoid or minimize it.

Bias refers to a distortion in the estimate of an effect measure—that is, it is higher or lower than it would be if we could obtain a less biased or unbiased estimate. In a cohort study, the effect measure of major interest is the relative risk. If a study is biased, the relative risk is higher or lower than it should be, and, if the distortion is large enough, this can lead to an erroneous inference about the importance of the relationship between a risk factor and a health outcome.

Long lists of potential sources of bias have been published (Feinstein, 1985; Sackett, 1979). Others have taken a more streamlined approach, subsuming the myriad sources of bias under major categories (Kleinbaum et al., 1982; Rothman, 1986). The latter approach will be used here. In the following sections, three major sources of bias will be discussed: selection, measurement, and confounding.

Selection Bias

Selection bias is a distortion in the estimate of effect resulting from the manner in which subjects are selected into the study population.

In a cohort study, potential sources of selection bias include (1) flaws in the choice of groups to be compared; (2) inability to locate or non-response of subjects selected into the sample resulting in differential effects on the comparison groups; and (3) because the design is longitudinal, subsequent attrition of subjects who had initially agreed to participate, which changes the composition of comparison groups. Knowledge of these likely sources of selection bias in a cohort study leads to two questions that can be used in the design, execution, reporting, and critique of such a study.

(1) *Are the cohorts that are being compared drawn from the same or similar populations?* A well-known source of selection bias, "the healthy worker effect," occurs when employed individuals are compared with those not employed (Fox & Collier, 1976; McMichael, 1976). Because individuals are selected in and out of the labor force on the basis of health status, employed people are healthier than the general population of the same age, race, and sex. Therefore, estimates of risk for adverse health outcomes based upon comparisons of employed groups with the general population are biased toward the null hypothesis. Waldron, Herold, Dunn, and Staum (1982) demonstrate empirically that this effect operates for women. In a study of the effects of women's roles on their health status as reflected in their reports of illness episodes in a health diary, Woods (1980) took steps to avoid this source of bias. She excluded from the analysis those women who were currently unable to work due to illness or injury, those who had been unable to work for more than six months due to the illness or injury, and those who had to change the kind or amount of work due to some illness or injury.

(2) *Has there been differential selection or loss to follow-up from the study groups?* In a follow-up or cohort study, the initial sample selection procedures are not as likely to introduce bias as is subsequent attrition of subjects during the follow-up period. In cross-sectional and case-comparison studies, a major issue is selective survival, that is, over- or underrepresentation of exposure among those who survive long enough to be selected into the sample. On the other hand, the major source of selection bias in a cohort study is subsequent attrition of subjects initially selected for study. The overall number of subjects lost is not as critical as the differential loss from study subgroups consisting of particular independent-dependent variable combinations, as illustrated in the following numerical example.

Assume that an investigator hypothesized that high exposure to a factor would be associated with increased incidence of a health problem. In her sample of 100 subjects, 50 were categorized as high on the exposure variable and 50 as low on this variable.

- *Scenario 1:* no attrition. If every subject remained in the study for the entire follow-up period of one year, and in each category of the independent variable 10 new cases of the health problem developed, the incidence rate would be 20% per year in each group. The relative risk would be 1.00, as shown in Table 10.2A.
- *Scenario 2:* loss of four subjects without differential loss from study subgroups. If one subject were lost from each of the four cells of the table, as illustrated in Table 10.2B, the incidence rate would be 18.75% in each group. Although this result differs from that obtained in the previous scenario, in which no attrition occurred, an unbiased estimate of effect is obtained. The relative risk is 1.00 because there has been no differential loss of subjects from the cells of the 2 × 2 table.
- *Scenario 3:* loss of four subjects with differential loss from study subgroups. If four subjects were lost from one of the four cells of the table, as illustrated in Table 10.2C, the incidence rate would be 20% per year in the exposed group and 13% per year in the unexposed group. The relative risk in this case is biased upward. It is 1.54 instead of 1.00, which it would have been had there been no differential attrition from the groups. This is how selection bias operates.

In summary, even the loss of a large percentage of subjects would not introduce bias unless the loss were distributed differentially as illustrated above. This assumes, of course, that there are still enough observations for statistical precision.

Measurement Bias

Measurement bias, sometimes referred to as information bias, occurs when the exposure variable (independent variable) or outcome (dependent variable) is measured in a way that is systematically inaccurate and results in distortion in the estimate of effect.

The major sources of measurement bias are (1) a defective measuring instrument, (2) a procedure for ascertaining the outcome that is not sufficiently sensitive and/or specific, (3) the likelihood of detecting the outcome dependent on exposure status, (4) selective recall of subjects, and (5) lack of blind measurements. See Kelsey et al. (1986, pp. 285-352) for an overview of measurement issues in epidemiology.

Table 10.2A Illustration of Selection Bias in a Cohort Study: Scenario 1, No Attrition

	Dependent Variable		
	Health Problem	*Health Problem*	
Independent Variable	*Develops*	*Does Not Develop*	*Total*
Exposed	10	40	50
Not exposed	10	40	50

NOTE: Incidence rate exposed group, 10/50 = .20 or 20 per 100 per year; incidence rate not exposed group, 10/50 = .20 or 20 per 100 per year; relative risk, .20/.20 = 1.00.

Table 10.2B Illustration of Selection Bias in a Cohort Study: Scenario 2, Loss of Four Subjects Without Differential Loss from Study Subgroups

	Dependent Variable		
	Health Problem	*Health Problem*	
Independent Variable	*Develops*	*Does Not Develop*	*Total*
Exposed	9	39	48
Not exposed	9	39	48

NOTE: Incidence rate exposed group, 9/48 = .1875 or 18.75 per 100 per year; incidence rate not exposed group, 9/48 = .1875 or 18.75 per 100 per year; relative risk, .1875/.1875 = 1.00.

Table 10.2C Illustration of Selection Bias in a Cohort Study: Scenario 3, Loss of Four Subjects with Differential Loss from Study Subgroups

	Dependent Variable		
	Health Problem	*Health Problem*	
Independent Variable	*Develops*	*Does Not Develop*	*Total*
Exposed	10	40	50
Not exposed	6	40	46

NOTE: Incidence rate exposed group, 10/50 = .20 or 20 per 100 per year; incidence rate not exposed group, 6/46 = .13 or 13 per 100 per year; relative risk, .20/.13 = 1.54.

Sensitivity and specificity. In the classic epidemiologic study, both the exposure and the outcome are categorical variables, very often a dichotomy. In this case, concurrent validity can be expressed as sensitivity, specificity, predictive value positive, and predictive value negative. In making a decision about the source of information to use and the methods of data collection, a methodological pilot study is in order to determine the best method when alternatives are available. A memorable example is provided by Lilienfeld and Graham (1958) in their study of the relationship between cervical cancer and circumcision of the partner. The decision was whether to determine circumcision status on the basis of physical exam or to rely on subject report of circumcision status. Obviously, the method used would make a great deal of difference in the facilities, time, personnel, and subject cooperation necessary for data collection. An empirical comparison of the two methods was undertaken to determine the accuracy of the self-report approach compared with the superior but more costly physical exam; the results are presented in Table 10.3.

The specificity indicates that a high percentage of those who were not circumcised (on the basis of physical exam) said that they were not (92.3%). Sensitivity was much lower; less than half of those who were circumcised reported that they were (43.2%). Predictive values indicate how well the subject's statement reflects actual circumcision status as categorized by physical exam. The predictive value positive indicates that a relatively high percentage of those who said they were circumcised actually were (86.4%). The predictive value of a negative statement was lower; of those who said they were not circumcised, only 59% were not, as indicated by physical exam.

The purpose of this type of analysis is to quantify the magnitude and describe the direction of bias in the measurement of a dichotomous variable. Further information can be obtained from epidemiology texts (e.g., Mausner & Kramer, 1985; Weiss, 1986). See Meininger (1985) for an illustration of its use in methodological research.

Blindness. In an observational design the investigator does not have control over the independent variables, so the issue of blindness in its manipulation is not relevant. What is extremely important in an observational study is blindness in the measurements. Subjects should not be alerted to the specific hypotheses being investigated. In the process of obtaining informed consent from subjects the researcher should be certain that they understand the nature of the data collection procedures that will be used. However, there are usually several groups of variables measured in addition to the independent and dependent variables, such as those that will be used to describe the sample and control variables. It is not advisable to alert subjects as to which ones are the key variables.

To maintain interviewer or observer blindness, the outcome should be measured without knowledge of the exposure status of the subject. This can be accomplished by using different data collectors for each

Table 10.3 Validity of Self-Reported Circumcision Status

| | Physical Exam | | |
Subject's Statement	Circumcised	Not Circumcised	Total
Circumcised	38	6	44
Not circumcised	50	72	122
Total	88	78	166

NOTE: Sensitivity = 38/88 × 100% = 43.2%; specificity = 72/78 × 100% = 92.3%; predictive value positive = 38/44 × 100% = 86.4%; predictive value negative = 72/122 × 100% = 59.0%.

set of variables and keeping them blind as to the status of the variable they are not measuring. Another approach that is often recommended is to keep data collectors blind as to the specific hypotheses under investigation.

Selective recall. The potential for selective or biased recall by subjects is not as great in a follow-up or cohort study as it is in a case-comparison study. This is because with the case-comparison approach, subjects are asked to recall their history of exposure after the outcome has already occurred. If the outcome has not yet occurred, as is the case in a prospective cohort study, the nature of the outcome cannot distort the reporting of the exposure. In a retrospective cohort study, the outcome has occurred at the time the data collection begins. However, the measurements of the independent variable were recorded previously and thus cannot be biased by the outcome (although they may be invalid or unreliable measurements for other reasons). Comparability of quality of information in the study subgroups should be a major consideration in planning data collection (MacMahon & Pugh, 1970, pp. 257-261). The circumstances of obtaining information from subjects (setting, length of interview, amount and content of probing) should be the same for all subjects. Although comparability can never be assured, the investigator can present evidence that there are no glaring differences between the groups. Noncomparability should be suspected if there are vastly different response rates for cases and controls (or exposed and unexposed subjects in a cohort study).

Confounding Bias

Confounding bias occurs when the exposure-outcome relationship under investigation is interrelated with an extraneous (or confounding) factor. Unless the confounding factor is controlled in the design of the study or in its analysis, distortion in the estimate of effect will result.

A confounding factor operates through its association with both the independent (exposure) and dependent (outcome) variables, producing an indirect statistical association.

In the planning phase of a research project, the investigator should identify factors that have the potential to confound the exposure-outcome relationship under investigation, and propose strategies for eliminating or controlling their effects. Knowledge of the subject matter and a thorough review of the literature are essential for the identification of these potentially confounding factors.

An important distinction between confounding bias and other types of bias is that confounding is correctable at the analysis stage, whereas selection and information biases are usually difficult if not impossible to correct at that stage. Confounding bias can be eliminated, controlled, or minimized at (1) the design stage by restricting the study sample to subjects with certain characteristics or by matching the comparison groups, and (2) at the analysis stage by using a multivariable approach to the statistical analysis to adjust for the confounding factors or by examining the exposure-outcome relationship within specified levels or categories of the confounding factor (stratified analysis).

A study by Woods (1980) illustrates control of potentially confounding variables by restriction of subject characteristics and by statistical analysis of data with multiple regression. The independent variables were role proliferation, sex role norm traditionalism, role reinforcement, and failure. The dependent variable was number of illness episodes as recorded in a health diary over a three-week period. Age, marital status, and source of health care were controlled by restricting the sample to married women between 20 and 40 years of age who were registrants at a particular family health clinic and lived within a 10-mile radius of it. At the analysis stage, multiple regression was used to examine the effects of the independent variables while controlling for other factors that could be correlated with number of illness episodes recorded: age, education, income, race, and number of children. Note that age was partially controlled at the design stage by restriction of the sample to those 20 to 40 years old. Any residual confounding due to age within this range was handled by adjusting for its effect statistically at the analysis stage.

Robarge, Reynolds, and Groothuis (1982) used sample restriction and matching to control for potentially confounding factors in their study of the relationship between twin births and child abuse. Sets of twins delivered at a specific hospital were included if their average birth weights exceeded 2,000 grams and if their five-minute apgars were greater than or equal to 6; 38 sets of twins met these criteria. Two or three single-birth infants who met the same criteria were individually matched to each set of twins for race, socioeconomic status, and maternal age. Although several differences between the characteristics of the twins and single births were noted by the authors, these variables were not evaluated for their confounding effects as reported in the article. If these other variables had confounding effects on the relationship under investigation, it would have been appropriate to control for them in the analysis.

Matching. Although matching is generally considered a powerful tool for achieving control in an experimental or observational study, it should be pointed out that a matched design has disadvantages as well as advantages. Matching is a very useful strategy for managing variables that would have a strong confounding effect. It is particularly useful in a small study in which there is little hope of controlling for the factor in the analysis because of lack of overlap between the study groups on the confounding factors.

A major disadvantage of matching is the time and effort it can take to find appropriate matches, particularly when several matching factors are specified and close matches are desired. Of course, the time and effort required to find appropriate matches depends on the size of the subject pool available and on access to information on variables that constitute selection criteria. If matching subjects are drawn from hospital records, a large pool of subjects and information about them may be readily available, provided access to the records is not a problem. On the other hand, if neighborhood controls are sought and several matching factors are involved, an extensive search may be necesary to find appropriate matches. A disadvantage of individual matching in a case-control study is that it precludes the ability to examine the effects of the matching factor. The implication is that a matching factor should be a well-known confounder, one that has been thoroughly demonstrated in previous studies. One should never match intervening variables, that is, those that are intermediate in the causal pathway between the risk factor and the disease (MacMahon & Pugh, 1970, p. 256). Matching on the intervening variable would eliminate the ability to detect a relationship between the risk factor and the disease.

A final caution about matching: There is a possibility of overmatching (MacMahon & Pugh, 1970, p. 256; Miettinen, 1985, p. 77; Schlesselman, 1982, p. 110). One can think of overmatching as a loss of efficiency. Recall that in a matched analysis, information for testing the hypothesis is gained only from discordant pairs. If there is a strong relationship between outcome status and the matching factor (in a case-control study), this overmatching will inflate the number of concordant pairs that are discarded from the analysis.

In considering the pros and cons of matching, the researcher should keep in mind that individual matching (or matched pairs, triplets, and so on) is not the only alternative. Frequency matching should also be considered. The goal of frequency matching is to achieve balance between the comparison groups in the proportion with or without given characteristics. If there are similar distributions of age, sex, and race in the comparison groups, the confounding effects of these variables are controlled.

TOWARD A STATISTICALLY RELIABLE STUDY: MINIMIZING CHANCE ERROR, MAXIMIZING POWER

The second aim of research design is to minimize random error in order to assure a reliable study, one that maximizes precision. Validity, the lack of systematic error, is of overriding concern to the researcher because a highly reliable but invalid study would yield a very precise estimate of the wrong answer. Assuming that a valid study is being designed, how would the researcher decide how large a sample is required to achieve statistical reliability? Sample size formulas and tables for epidemiologic studies are available (Schlesselman, 1974, 1982; Walter, 1977). These formulas relate the size of the sample to the following elements (Rothman, 1986):

(1) level of statistical significance (alpha error)
(2) chance of missing a real effect (beta error)
(3) magnitude of effect
(4) disease rate in the absence of exposure (or exposure prevalence in the absence of disease)
(5) relative size of the compared groups (i.e., ratio of cases to controls)

Holding everything else constant, the power of a study can be increased by increasing the sample size.

A major advantage of a case-control design over a cohort design is the number of subjects required. Schlesselman (1982) provides the following illustration of a study designed to determine whether maternal exposure to estrogens around the time of conception results in an increased risk of congenital heart defects among offspring. If 8 heart defects occurred per 1,000 births among unexposed women, a cohort study would require observation of the pregnancy outcomes of 3,889 women exposed to estrogens and 3,889 unexposed women in order to detect a relative risk of 2.0 or greater. A case-control study would require only 188 cases and 188 controls if approximately 30% of women were exposed to estrogens around the time of conception. If one were interested in a specific heart defect that occurred at a rate of 2 cases per 1,000 births, a cohort study would require follow-up on approximately 15,700 women exposed to estrogens and 15,700 women not exposed in order to detect a twofold or greater increase in risk. The case-control approach would require only 188 cases and 188 controls. This illustration points out the advantages of a case-control study in terms of sample size, particularly for studying outcomes that occur rarely.

Keep in mind that sample size estimates are not nearly as accurate as they appear. They are based on figures that are "estimates"—more accurately described as "guesses." Furthermore, the simplest formulas do not take into account design and analysis nuances such as confounding, interaction, nonresponse, subgroup analysis, and matching.

HUMAN SUBJECTS ISSUES

Epidemiologic design issues that have the potential to impinge on the rights of human subjects are similar to those encountered in other types of research. An issue that has particular relevance to the design of epidemiologic studies is the use of records to define a population from which to sample or to find particular types of subjects.

CAUSAL INFERENCES BASED ON EPIDEMIOLOGIC EVIDENCE

One of the major aims of epidemiologic research is to study the etiology of disease. Implicit in this aim is the need to infer cause-and-effect relationships. Because epidemiologists often investigate problems that cannot be studied experimentally with human subjects and because animal models are not always appropriate, rigorous observational designs are the specialty of the epidemiologist. Rarely is there certainty about the link between a putative cause and an adverse health outcome. Rather, risk factors are studied in relation to the probability of a specified change in health status.

In addition to critiquing the internal and external validity of each individual study, the following criteria are used to review, evaluate, and synthesize findings from more than one study on the same topic (Hill, 1965, 1971).

(1) *The strength of the association:* The magnitude of an effect is used in evaluating the strength of an association. The measure of effect in most epidemiologic studies is the relative risk. It is more difficult to find alternative explanations for strong associations. Note that a probability value does not convey information about the strength of an association; a very weak relationship can be highly statistically significant if the sample size is large enough.

(2) *Dose-response effect:* An increasing frequency of disease with an increasing level of exposure to the risk factor (dose) points toward a causal association, but there may be alternative explanations for this finding (Weiss, 1981). On the other hand, its absence is not evidence against a causal association. For instance, a causal relationship may take the form of a threshhold effect rather than a dose-response effect.

(3) *Lack of temporal ambiguity:* The risk factor must precede the development of the outcome. For instance, if an association is observed between depression and chronic illness, one could not consider depression a risk factor unless it preceded the occurrence of the disease. In other words, a purported risk factor must be identifiable as an antecedent to the outcome rather than a consequence.

(4) *Consistency:* If findings are replicated, this is good evidence for a causal association, but it is neither necessary nor sufficient evidence. Lack of consistency may be due to differences in methods and samples, and to secular changes. On the other hand, consistent results may be found in several studies that are biased in the same direction.

(5) *Coherence of the evidence:* This means that the results are not inconsistent with known facts. However, ignorance about a problem may impede the ability to evaluate inconsistencies.

(6) *Biological plausibility:* This evidence is helpful, but an association may be judged to be causal before we have enough knowledge to state how the cause leads to the effect. In meeting this criterion, we often need to rely on laboratory studies of disease models in order to understand the pathways through which the risk factor operates.

(7) *Specificity of the association:* This criterion implies that a risk factor is associated with only one disease, and/or a disease is associated with one risk factor. Specificity is not usually an appropriate criterion because most health outcomes have multiple causes and many risk factors have multiple effects.

These criteria should be used as guidelines for organizing evidence of causality rather than as a checklist. A recent example is provided by Matthews and Haynes (1986). This discussion serves only as an introduction to views held by some epidemiologists. The reader is referred to the following references for more extensive background on the topic: Evans (1976, 1978), Lilienfeld and Lilienfeld (1980), MacMahon and Pugh (1970), Susser (1973).

SUMMARY

Experimental and observational designs are used in epidemiology, although the emphasis is on observational approaches. Even when an experimental design is employed in an epidemiologic study, it is usually carried out in an uncontrolled environment. Because experimentation is not always an ethical or feasible approach to studying health outcomes in human populations, epidemiologists have developed and adopted rigorous observational approaches in order to control the myriad sources of bias that can invalidate the study of naturally occurring events.

The emphasis in this chapter has been on cohort designs. Studies with cohort design features are much more prevalent in the nursing literature than are case-comparison studies. The major advantage of a cohort study is that subjects are observed for the occurrence of the outcome. Thus the risk factor can be identified as an antecedent to the outcome rather than as a consequence. The major advantage of a case-comparison study is in the much smaller sample size required. If carefully designed and executed, this can be a very powerful approach.

Three sources of bias that could threaten the internal validity of an epidemiologic study have been discussed: selection, measurement, and confounding. Approaches to avoiding or adjusting for these biases have been delineated. Finally, guidelines for drawing causal inferences from epidemiologic data were presented.

REFERENCES

Ballard, S., & McNamara, R. (1983). Quantifying nursing needs in home health care. *Nursing Research, 32,* 236-241.

Elandt-Johnson, R. C. (1975). Definition of rates: Some remarks on their use and misuse. *American Journal of Epidemiology, 102,* 267-271.

Evans, A. S. (1976). Causation and disease: The Henle-Koch postulates revisited. *Yale Journal of Biology and Medicine, 49,* 175-195.

Evans, A. S. (1978). Causation and disease: A chronological journey. *American Journal of Epidemiology, 108,* 249-258.

Feinstein, A. R. (1985). *Clinical epidemiology: The architecture of clinical research.* Philadelphia: W. B. Saunders.

Fleiss, J. L. (1981). *Statistical methods for rates and proportions.* New York: John Wiley.

Fox, A. J., & Collier, P. F. (1976). Low mortality rates in industrial cohort studies due to selection for work and survival in the industry. *British Journal of Preventive and Social Medicine, 30,* 225-230.

Francis, T. J., Korns, R. F., Voight, R. B., Biosen, M., Hemphill, F. M., Napier, J. A., & Tolchinsky, E. (1955). An evaluation of the 1954 poliomyelitis vaccine trials: Summary report. *American Journal of Public Health, 45,* 1-63.

Hill, A. B. (1965). The environment and disease: Association or causation? *Proceedings of the Royal Society of Medicine, 58,* 295-300.

Hill, A. B. (1971). *Principles of medical statistics* (9th ed.). New York: Oxford University Press.

Jacobsen, B. S., & Meininger, J. C. (1985). Designs and methods of published nursing research: 1956-1983. *Nursing Research, 34,* 306-312.

Jones, C. (1981). Father to infant attachment: Effects of early contact and characteristics of the infant. *Research in Nursing and Health, 4,* 193-200.

Kelsey, J. L., Thompson, W. D., & Evans, A. S. (1986). *Methods in observational epidemiology.* New York: Oxford University Press.

Kleinbaum, D. G., Kupper, L. L., & Morgenstern, H. (1982). *Epidemiologic methods: Principles and quantitative methods.* Belmont, CA: Wadsworth.

Lilienfeld, A. M., & Graham, S. (1958). Validity of determining circumcision status by questionnaire as related to epidemiological studies of cancer of the cervix. *Journal of the National Cancer Institute, 21,* 713-720.

Lilienfeld, A. M., & Lilienfeld, D. E. (1980). *Foundations of epidemiology.* New York: Oxford University Press.

MacMahon, B., & Pugh, T. F. (1970). *Epidemiology: Principles and methods.* Boston: Little, Brown.

Matthews, K. A., & Haynes, S. G. (1986). Type A behavior pattern and coronary disease risk: Update and critical evaluation. *American Journal of Epidemiology, 123,* 923-960.

Mausner, J. S., & Kramer, S. (1985). *Epidemiology: An introductory text* (2nd ed.). Philadelphia: W. B. Saunders.

McMichael, A. J. (1976). Standardized mortality ratios and the "healthy worker effect": Scratching beneath the surface. *Journal of Occupational Medicine, 18,* 165-168.

Meininger, J. C. (1985). Validity of Type A behavior scales for employed women. *Journal of Chronic Diseases, 38,* 375-383.

Miettinen, O. S. (1985). *Theoretical epidemiology: Principles of occurrence research in medicine.* New York: John Wiley.

Multiple Risk Factor Intervention Trial Group. (1982). Multiple Risk Factor Intervention

Trial: Risk factor changes and mortality results. *Journal of the American Medical Association, 248,* 1465-1477.

Norbeck, J. S., & Tilden, V. P. (1983). Life stress, social support and emotional disequilibrium in complications of pregnancy: A prospective multivariate study. *Journal of Health and Social Behavior, 24,* 30-46.

Robarge, J. P., Reynolds, Z. B., & Groothuis, J. R. (1982). Increased child abuse in families with twins. *Research in Nursing and Health, 5,* 199-203.

Rothman, K. J. (1986). *Modern epidemiology.* Boston: Little, Brown.

Sackett, D. L. (1979). Bias in analytic research. *Journal of Chronic Diseases, 32,* 51-63.

Schlesselman, J. J. (1974). Sample size requirements in cohort and case-control studies of disease. *American Journal of Epidemiology, 99,* 381-384.

Schlesselman, J. J. (1982). *Case-control studies: Design, conduct and analysis.* New York: Oxford University Press.

Susser, M. (1973). *Causal thinking in the health sciences: Concepts and strategies in epidemiology.* New York: Oxford University Press.

Waldron, I., Herold, J., Dunn, D., & Staum, R. (1982). Reciprocal effects of health and labor force participation among women: Evidence from two longitudinal studies. *Journal of Occupational Medicine, 24,* 126-132.

Walter, S. D. (1977). Determination of significant relative risks and optimal sampling procedures in prospective and retrospective comparative studies of various sizes. *American Journal of Epidemiology, 105,* 387-397.

Weiss, N. S. (1981). Inferring causal relationships: Elaboration of the criterion of "dose-response." *American Journal of Epidemiology, 113,* 487-490.

Weiss, N. S. (1986). *Clinical epidemiology: The study of the outcome of illness.* New York: Oxford University Press.

Woods, N. F. (1980). Women's roles and illness episodes: A prospective study. *Research in Nursing and Health, 3,* 137-145.

ADDITIONAL READINGS

Textbooks and Study Guides

Fletcher, R. H., Fletcher, S. W., & Wagner, E. H. (1987). *Clinical epidemiology: The essentials.* Baltimore: Williams & Wilkins.

Friedman, G. D. (1987). *Primer of epidemiology* (3rd ed.). New York: McGraw-Hill.

Hennekens, C. II., & Buring, J. E. (1987). *Epidemiology in medicine.* Boston: Little, Brown.

Morton, R. F., & Hebel, J. R. (1984). *A study guide to epidemiology and statistics.* Rockville, MD: Aspen.

Sackett, D. L., Haynes, R. B., & Tugwell, P. (1985). *Clinical epidemiology: A basic science for clinical medicine.* Boston: Little, Brown.

Slome, C., Brogan, D., Eyres, S., & Lednar, W. (1982). *Basic epidemiological methods and biostatistics: A workbook.* Monterey, CA: Wadsworth Health Sciences.

Designing Observational Studies

Cole, P. (1979). The evolving case-control study. *Journal of Chronic Diseases, 32,* 15-27.

Copeland, K. T., Checkoway, H., McMichael, A. J., & Holbrook, R. H. (1977). Bias due to misclassification in the estimation of relative risk. *American Journal of Epidemiology, 105,* 488-495.

Feinleib, M. (1987). Biases and weak associations. *Preventive Medicine, 16,* 150-164.

Feinstein, A. R. (1985). Experimental requirements and scientific principles in case-control studies. *Journal of Chronic Diseases, 38,* 127-133.

Freeman, J., & Hutchinson, G. B. (1980). Prevalence, incidence and duration. *American Journal of Epidemiology, 112,* 707-723.

Greenland, S. (1977). Response and follow-up bias in cohort studies. *American Journal of Epidemiology, 106,* 184-187.

Hartge, P., Brinton, L. A., Rosenthal, J. F., Cahill, J. I., Hoover, R. M., & Waksberg, J. (1984). Random digit dialing in selecting a population-based control group. *American Journal of Epidemiology, 120,* 825-833.

Hayden, G. F., Kramer, M. S., & Horwitz, R. I. (1982). The case-control study: A practical review for the clinician. *Journal of the American Medical Association, 247,* 326-331.

Kalish, L. A., & Begg, C. D. (1987). Evaluation of efficient designs for observational epidemiologic studies. *Biometrics, 43,* 145-167.

Kramer, M. S., & Boivin, J. F. (1987). Toward an "unconfounded" classification of epidemiologic research design. *Journal of Chronic Diseases, 40,* 683-688.

McKinley, S. M. (1977). Pair matching: A reappraisal of a popular technique. *Biometrics, 33,* 725-735.

Miettinen, O. S. (1970). Matching and design efficiency in retrospective studies. *American Journal of Epidemiology, 91,* 111-117.

Nair, R. C. (1984). Statistical problems associated with cohort studies of workers in an industry. *Annals Academy of Medicine, 13* (suppl.), 317-320.

Schlesselman, J. J. (1974). Sample size requirements in cohort and case-control studies of disease. *American Journal of Epidemiology, 99,* 381-384.

Spitzer, W. O. (1985). Ideas and words: Two dimensions for debates on case controlling. *Journal of Chronic Diseases, 38,* 541-542.

Szklo, M. (1987). Design and conduct of epidemiologic studies. *Preventive Medicine, 16,* 142-149.

Thompson, W. D., Kelsey, J. L., & Walter, S. D. (1982). Cost and efficiency in the choice of matched and unmatched study designs. *American Journal of Epidemiology, 116,* 840-851.

Walter, S. D. (1976). The estimation and interpretation of attributable risk in health research. *Biometrics, 32,* 829-849.

Designing Clinical Trials

Chalmers, T., Smith, H., Blackburn, B., Silverman, B., Schroeder, B., Reitman, D., & Ambroz, A. (1981). A method for assessing the quality of a randomized control trial. *Controlled Clinical Trials, 2,* 31-49.

Ellenberg, S. S. (1984). Randomization designs in comparative clinical trials. *New England Journal of Medicine, 310,* 1404-1408.

Friedman, L. M., Furberg, C. D., & DeMets, D. L. (1985). *Fundamentals of clinical trials* (2nd ed.). Littleton, MA: PSG.

Frieman, J. A., Chalmers, T. C., Smith, H., Jr., & Kuebler, R. (1978). The importance of beta, the type II error and sample size in the design and interpretation of the randomized control trial: Survey of 71 "negative" trials. *New England Journal of Medicine, 299,* 690-694.

Meinert, C. (1986). *Clinical trials.* New York: Oxford University Press.

Mosteller, F., Gilbert, J. P., & McPeek, B. (1980). Reporting standards and research strategies for controlled trials: Agenda for the editor. *Controlled Clinical Trials, 1,* 37-58.

Pocock, S. J. (1983). *Clinical trials: A practical approach.* Chichester: John Wiley.

Pocock, S. J. (1985). Current issues in the design and interpretation of clinical trials. *British Medical Journal, 296,* 39-42.

11. Evaluative Designs

Marilynn J. Wood

Evaluative research designs are intended to provide data on the success of action programs. They are of particular interest to policymakers who are responsible for allocating resources in health care. In nursing, we are frequently called upon to design program evaluations for many reasons, ranging from developing grant proposals for training or clinical projects to testing the effectiveness of nursing intervention programs in the clinical setting. The value of evaluation has become increasingly apparent to politicians and granting agencies for budget appropriations and funding of programs. In addition, within health care agencies evaluative research is becoming an important management tool, used to determine whether individual programs are producing benefits that justify their costs.

These research designs do not fit into any one level of research, but instead usually have characteristics of more than one level. They are based on the objectives of the program, and therefore may combine several designs into one. Evaluation uses the methods and tools of research but applies them in an action setting that may not always fit with the assumptions and principles of traditional research. To conduct evaluation research, we need to be aware of the differences between using research principles for evaluative purposes and using them for projects that are strictly research endeavors.

Evaluative designs are appropriate whenever the research question asks about the effectiveness of a program. For example, the researcher might be interested in whether or not a cardiac rehabilitation program really has an effect on the health and future productivity of the participants, and whether or not the cost of the program can be justified in terms of the results. This is a typical evaluative research question. The question could be partially answered using an experimental design, with randomly assigned groups. However, an experimental design would be very expensive and would not make use of existing resources (such as a cardiac rehabilitation program already operating in the community). Requiring a control group and random assignment to groups might be unethical if a rehabilitation program is already established. In addition, it is difficult to assess long-range effects (including cost-benefit ratios) through the standard experimental design because of the influence of time on the outcome. Finally, the experimental design is always implemented in an artificial setting, and so may not provide an adequate test of the real-life situation. An evaluative design can incorporate some of the control techniques of an experimental design while utilizing both survey and qualitative methods to provide additional data. Its main purpose, however, is to *measure the effects* of the program.

Difficulties may arise in planning evaluative research, stemming largely from the fact that the programs being evaluated are so variable. In health care, the range of programs that need to be evaluated is vast, ranging from small, self-learning modules for teaching students to calculate dosages to complex programs designed to change the image of nursing in the eyes of the general public. There are various factors related to the program itself that will affect the evaluative approach that can be taken. These relate, first, to the scope of the program itself in terms of the geographic area affected and the size of the population served by the program. Second, the quality of the program goals will be a significant factor. Can these be explained easily, in precise terms, or are they vague and global in nature? Certainly, goals that are clearly stated in measurable terms will simplify the approach that can be taken, whereas more diffuse goals will require a different approach. Finally, the innovativeness of the approach taken in the program will be a determining factor in the approach that can be taken for evaluation.

In addition to these program factors, however, the politics of evaluation must be kept in mind (Borg & Gall, 1983). In any program, there will be various individuals and groups who have vested interest in the program, and who may try to influence the evaluation accordingly. The reality of the situation is that an evaluation can sometimes do more harm than good, particularly if people feel threatened by the evaluation and their job performance is adversely affected. By including these stakeholders in planning the evaluation, the researcher can include their concerns and issues in the plan and many potential problems can be diffused.

Assumptions of the Design

The following assumptions are implicit in the use of evaluative designs:

(1) There are measurable objectives for the program that can be used as a basis for evaluation.
(2) There are methods or tools available with which to measure the variables.
(3) The objectives can be assigned priorities and weighted in a practical sense according to their value to the project.
(4) Adequate control subjects can be provided so that a model for statistical testing can be used to establish whether or not the program made a difference.

Basic Design

The question being asked in an evaluative study is, What difference did the program make? The first step in setting up the design is to specify the objectives of the program in measurable terms (Cain & Hollister, 1972). This may have been done when the program was initiated, but it is unlikely that it was if the program was set up as a clinical or social program. Patton (1980) suggests having the program directors develop a set of evaluation questions based on what they would like to know about the results of the program. These questions or objectives must then be listed in order of priority. The process may involve moving from an extensive list of potential questions to a much shorter list of relevant questions to a "focused list of essential and necessary questions" (Patton, 1980, p. 96). Next, a priority list is developed that demonstrates the importance of each objective in relation to the overall mission of the program. For example, for a program designed to provide posthospitalization follow-up care for hypertensives, the primary objective should relate to the actual blood pressure of the participants and how well it is maintained within the normal range for each individual. The attitudes of the participants and their families toward the program, although important to measure, would be given lower priority because they are not directly related to the central mission of the program. Methods of measuring the achievement of the objectives must be demonstrated. If any of the major objectives are intangible in nature, the researcher may recommend qualitative methods for the measurement of these objectives. Once the objectives have been formulated and priorities decided, an appropriate control group must be established. In this respect, the design will usually resemble a quasi-experimental design.

The ideal evaluative design has the major ingredients of an experimental design, but there is one important difference: Because the study is evaluating a specific program, the program participants usually constitute the "experimental" subjects, rather than a sample of individuals chosen specifically for a research project. This is an important distinction because the selection of these participants is usually determined by the program protocol, not by the researcher. Therefore, they are not randomly assigned and there is no assurance of equivalence between experimental and control subjects. Cain and Hollister (1972) suggest the following possible alternative methods for obtaining control group data:

(1) *Nonequivalent controls.* Controls may be a sample of individuals not participating in the program, but are matched with program participants on some significant demographic variables. Although such a matched group can serve as a viable control group, it is likely to be somewhat nonrepresentative; that is, it may differ significantly from the program participant group in some critical ways. It is sometimes possible to construct a control group from persons who have the same disease process as program participants, but who have chosen an alternate method of treatment. In this situation, control subjects would likely be very similar to the program participants, leading to a significant increase in the internal validity of the study. In other cases, however, the control subjects might be persons who were eligible for but chose not to participate in any program of treatment, and thus may resemble the participants only in one basic characteristic, such as diagnosis.

An alternative to the matched control group is a large-scale control group from the target population. In this case, the sheer size of the control group increases the validity of the study by ensuring that relevant variables are normally distributed. Large-scale control groups can be randomly selected from the population, thus yielding a sample representative of the population. However, because the program participants are chosen selectively rather than randomly, the unavoidable occurrence of unmeasured variables among experimental subjects makes it difficult to compare them to the control group. This problem might prove serious enough to render this type of control group invalid. If so, a matched group will provide a better comparison than a large-scale group.

(2) *The before-and-after design.* In this design, each subject is expected to be his or her own control. Specifically, a baseline measurement taken on each individual before implementation of the program is used to determine how these persons would perform if there were no program. This method, of course, gives no assurance of internal validity. Numerous factors other than the program itself could be responsible for any changes observed in the participants. In many situations, one would expect the subjects to undergo change irrespective of treatment programs. These anticipated changes, which can reflect either improvement (as in a rehabilitation program) or deterioration (as in a hospice program), can make it impossible to identify the impact of the program itself when subjects are used as their own controls.

In addition, other changes in the lives of the particpants can occur that have nothing to do with the program but that affect any before-and-after comparison. This design, therefore, should be reserved for use with groups for which the "without treatment" course of events for the subjects is well documented and predictable, thus increasing the possibility of internal validity for the study.

(3) *Alternative experimental designs.* Boruch and Wortman (1979) discuss ways to couple randomized experiments with evaluative studies that try to approximate experiments through the use of statistical analysis. Specifically the evaluative design can incorporate statistical techniques that approximate randomization—and yield comparison groups that are similar to the program population.

It is quite possible, in an evaluation study, that the measurement techniques might involve both quantitative and qualitative data. Qualitative data, such as participant observation, in-depth interviewing, and detailed description, can be of great help to the evaluative researcher in providing a richness of background that puts the data into the context of the participants and the program itself. It can also be of great value in analyzing and interpreting the quantitative data. For example, when analyzing data about dropouts from a particular program, instead of merely interpreting the numbers in light of the demographic characteristics of dropouts versus continuers, it can be very enlightening to have descriptive data on the feelings and perceptions of the participants including their reasons for either staying with the program or dropping out. In fact, an evaluative design that does not include some of these data would be subject to suspicion. Because the design mimics but does not equal the experimental design, it can be tempting to analyze and interpret the results *as though it were a true experiment*. The inclusion of qualitative data prevents this from happening, as the quantitative analysis must then be discussed in light of the qualitative data.

Variations on the Basic Design

An interesting variation on the traditional evaluative design is seen in the case of the *needs assessment*. This type of evaluative research is very important because it puts program design in touch with the realities of the health care system and the consumer. A well-designed needs assessment will also indicate any need to change existing programs.

A needs assessment will normally be designed as a survey, using a questionnaire that collects data from respondents on both the existing and the desired situation (see Chapter 6, on descriptive designs). By defining a need as "a discrepancy between an existing set of conditions and a desired set of conditions," Borg and Gall (1983, p. 753) recommend that a needs assessment be viewed as a discrepancy analysis of current and desired conditions. This sounds quite simple and straightforward, but there are some issues with regard to needs assessments that should be addressed.

One of these relates to the values underlying needs. These may not be addressed by the assessment tool. For example, Dela Cruz, Jacobs, and Wood (1986) surveyed home health agencies in Southern California to determine the learning needs of home health nurses. The survey items elicited information about the existing educational background of home health nurses and about perceived need for additional knowledge in a variety of areas. The resultant data provided the basis for a continuing education program for these nurses. The questionnaire did not, however, address the underlying values of the participants. Participants might differ in how they believe educational deficits among home health nurses should be addressed. Some might believe that a continuing education program is not appropriate for nurses who are not adequately prepared to practice home health nursing, and that these nurses should be required to obtain bachelor's degrees instead.

Another issue regarding needs assessments stems from the fact that the results are pooled and reported as group trends. Important individual differences can be overlooked, and this could cause problems when a program is implemented.

Examples of Evaluative Studies

Martinson et al. (1986) evaluated a home care alternative to hospital care for children dying of cancer. The program provided care to 64 children referred by oncologists and pediatricians in the north central United States. The children were 17 years of age or younger and dying of cancer. Hospitalization was not planned at time of referral. The design did not include a control group; rather, the progress of each child was evaluated on the basis of the program objectives. The major objective was to allow the child to die at home.

Data were collected from medical records, home care records, questionnaires covering demographic data, grief support lists, care ratings, and progress recordings made by the project nurse coordinators. A one-month postdeath interview with parents reviewed the process of home care and parent assessment of care, as well as financial aspects of the care. Another interview was conducted one year after the child's death.

The home care program successfully provided care to 58 families, 46 of whom experienced the death of a child at home. At one-month and one-year intervals after the child's death, the 46 families expressed satisfaction with the experience. This evaluative design is typical in that neither the internal nor the external validity of the design is documented, yet the project objectives are supported.

In a different type of evaluative study, Thurston and Dundas (1985) looked at the effectiveness of an early postpartum discharge program in a large Canadian city. Two major hospitals and the city home care program participated in the study. The major purpose of the program was to provide a safe alternative to hospital care for postpartum patients. Patient safety and satisfaction were high-priority objectives for the project. The program participants were volunteers (both mothers and physicians) who met elaborate admission criteria ensuring that there were no complications related to the delivery. The program was begun as a pilot study with 109 patients, and was continued over 7 months for an additional 267 patients. No control group was established, due to the fact that postpartum complications that might be prevented by longer hospitalization are well documented. Measurements were established for critical areas of patient safety, including PKU testing of infants, necessity of hospital readmission, and complications for either mother or infant. Patient satisfaction was measured through the use of a questionnaire, for which a return rate of 69% was achieved.

The results demonstrated that the two central objectives of the program were met, in that there were no serious complications for mothers and infants that were attributable to early discharge, and the subjects expressed satisfaction with the program. Limitations of the design were acknowledged, including the self-selecting, voluntary nature of the subjects. As frequently happens with evaluation studies, the positive results led to the incorporation of the program into the routine service of the community prior to the anticipated end of the evaluation study.

Suitable Nursing Problems

Evaluative designs are the best choice for many nursing situations. An evaluative design might even be required, particularly for programs funded by external granting agencies. In these cases, the evaluation must be planned as part of the program. In addition to these mandated evaluations, however, the design can be used by nurses to study phenomena that would otherwise be impossible to study without extensive funding. The evaluative design, unlike the experimental design, can utilize existing programs and test the effectiveness of various interventions without having to set up special treatment programs. The design could be used, for example, to test the effectiveness with which a weight-loss program prepares individuals to maintain their weight loss, the preparedness for bereavement of families of hospice patients, the readiness of graduates of rehabilitation programs to resume product lives, or the professional socialization of students in nursing programs. The criterion for selecting an evaluative design is that the research question be part of the program objectives. If it is, then the evaluative design is appropriate. If not, another design should be selected.

A useful distinction can be made between *formative* and *summative* evaluation. Formative evaluation provides feedback during the progress of the program and is used to improve or modify its operation. Summative evaluation is done after the program is over and attempts to assess how effective the program was in meeting its objectives. Although some programs make use of both types, evaluative research is primarily concerned with summative evaluation (Cain & Hollister, 1972).

The first step in designing an evaluation study is to state the program goals clearly. This can prove to be the most difficult step in the process. For evaluation purposes, the goals must be stated in measurable terms. Thus the process is enhanced if the researcher assists the project staff to formulate clear, specific, and measurable goals in the development phase of the project. Otherwise, the program goals may be extremely fuzzy, and the staff might not reach a consensus as to what the program is trying to do. The researcher can either work collaboratively with the staff to define the programs's goals or formulate goals unilaterally and present them to the staff. In either case, a consensus must be reached. If the views of the staff are extremely diverse, a preliminary exploratory study can be undertaken to describe what the various components of the program are doing; content analysis can then be used to formulate specific objectives for the program.

Once the goals are defined, the investigator must decide which of them to use for evaluation. A priority model can be used to determine which objectives are critical to the program and which are secondary. Although secondary objectives may be easier to measure, the evaluative researcher must first attempt to study the vital goals of the project and not be distracted by interesting but minor concerns. Once the vital goals are identified, some measurable indicators of success must be developed. These outcome criteria will be critically important to the success of the evaluation.

The major concern with evaluative designs is internal validity. We have already discussed how the assignment of subjects to treatment and control groups can compromise internal validity. Just as important, however, are problems with external validity. These concerns arise because the design does not require random sampling of subjects, thus creating a potential for selection bias. Sample selection in evaluative research is much more likely to be purposive than random; therefore, the researcher is faced with accounting for possible bias introduced in the selection process. One possible source of bias is self-selection (Bernstein, 1976). Many health care programs are available to the public on a self-selection basis. In this case, the target population must be defined as those who choose to participate in the program. For example, the success of a health screening program designed to identify persons at risk for heart disease and refer them for preventive care cannot be generalized to the entire population of potential heart disease patients. Even if the persons at risk were randomly assigned to different treatment programs, the relative effectiveness of each treatment could be generalized only to those persons who sought health screening. It is tempting to plan programs for the whole population based on the results of evaluation studies, paricularly when the demonstrated effects are tremendously successful. However, one cannot assume that persons who voluntarily seek health care from a particular program are indeed representative of the population at large. Only random sampling from the larger population will produce truly generalizable results, but replication of the study with different groups will increase our confidence in the results.

When selecting a program to evaluate, the researcher will frequently choose the one that is thought to be producing the best results. Similarly, in order to demonstrate that a program is ineffective, a poorly operated program might be chosen. In this way, the likelihood of obtaining usable results is enhanced. However, this process introduces selection bias. When an exceptionally good program is chosen, the results resemble those of an experimental design in that the researcher has maximized internal validity by eliminating many potential sources of error that might occur in programs less well operated. However, the ability to generalize the positive outcome to other such programs may be limited. This limitation must be recognized when presenting the results. Table 11.1, from Patton (1980) provides an excellent reference for the various types of sampling used in evaluation studies and the key issues accompanying each type.

Table 11.1 Sampling Issues in Evaluative Designs

Type	*Purpose*
(A) Random sampling	Avoids systematic bias in the sample; large sample size important for making generalizations
(1) simple random sample	Achieve a representative sample that permits generalizations to the whole population
(2) stratified random cluster samples	Increase confidence in making generalizations to particular subgroups or areas.
(B) Purposeful sampling	Increase utility of information obtained in small samples; sampling criteria based on the reputation of programs among key decision makers and/or on previous data collected from programs
(1) sampling extreme or deviant cases	Provide decision makers with information about unusual cases that may be particularly troublesome or enlightening, e.g., outstanding successes/notable failures; program with long waiting lists vs. programs with recruitment problems; unusually high morale and low morale problems, etc.
(2) sampling typical cases	Avoid studying a program where the results would be dismissed outright because *that* program is known to be special, deviant, unusual, extreme, etc.
(3) maximum variation sampling— picking three or four cases that represent a range on some dimension (e.g., size, location, budget)	Increase confidence in common patterns that cut across different programs; document unique program variations that have emerged in adapting to different conditions.
(4) sampling critical cases	Permits *logical* generalization and maximum application of information to other cases because if it's true in this one case, it's likely to be true of all other cases.
(5) sampling politically important or sensitive cases	Attracts attention to the study (or avoids attracting undesired attention by purposefully eliminating from the sample politically sensitive cases).
(6) convenience sampling —take the easy cases	Saves time, money and effort.

SOURCE: Patton (1980). Qualitative Evaluation Methods. Beverly Hills, CA: Sage.

DATA ANALYSIS

Data analysis has received considerable attention in evaluation studies that use nonexperimental and quasi-experimental designs.

Criticism of these designs usually revolves around internal validity (Alwin & Sullivan, 1976). Because randomization is not feasible in most cases, the possibility always exists that the experimental and control groups were not equivalent prior to the start of the program and that these differences have seriously affected the dependent variable.

In designs that incorporate at least one "experimental" group and one control group, an analysis of variance (ANOVA) would normally be used to look for significant differences among the groups. However, because the absence of equivalence among groups in evaluative designs compromises internal validity, ANOVA will not give an accurate picture of those differences. Alwin and Sullivan (1976) recommend that a special form of regression analysis be used to identify pretreatment differences on variables known to be relevant causes of the major outcome measure for the program. When significant pretreatment differences on any of these variables are found, a covariance analysis can hold constant the effects of one or more significant covariates so that the effect of the program on the outcome criterion can be estimated.

When qualitative data have been collected as part of the design, content analysis will be required as part of the analytic process. When performing content analysis on data from control and experimental subjects, the researcher should take care that the analysis is done without knowledge of which subjects were in the control and which were in the experimental group. The groups can then be compared on the categorizations that were found in the data, in addition to any statistical analysis that has been done.

RELIABILITY AND VALIDITY

Since measurement error jeopardizes both internal and external validity, and these two concepts are already compromised in an evaluative design, it becomes critical that the instruments be well designed and highly reliable, so that validity can be maximized. It follows, therefore, that the key objectives of the program must be stated in measurable terms, and that the outcome criteria must be easily quantifiable. This is not always easily achieved in evaluative research, since some of the objectives may be vague and difficult to quantify. In this case, employing multiple means of assessment will strengthen the design. The collection of qualitative data can strengthen (or weaken) confidence in the validity of the instruments by providing the perspective of the participants without the restriction of any particular point of view.

ETHICAL ISSUES

The issues surrounding the rights of human subjects in evaluative designs are similar to those involved with experimental designs. The ethical treatment of control groups is of concern, especially when a control group may be randomly selected from among program participants. In this case, informed consent must be obtained from the control subjects and they must be given the opportunity to benefit from the program itself once the data are collected.

Informed consent, in particular free informed consent, is the key issue for all subjects in evaluative studies. Usually the experimental subjects have voluntarily sought out the program and have not been recruited by the researcher. They have volunteered for an action program, not for a research project. In funded demonstration projects, however, all program applicants are commonly required to take part in the evaluation study. This can be construed as a form of coercion. Because public money funds these programs, it is generally deemed acceptable for subjects to be asked to participate in the evaluation as their contribution to the public good. Participation may thus be viewed as a form of payment for the benefit they will receive from the program. Nevertheless, subjects must clearly understand that they will be research subjects as well as program participants, and their rights to confidentiality and anonymity must be protected. In this area, evaluation research differs appreciably from other types of research because the primary emphasis is on the program rather than the research.

RESEARCH PROPOSAL

In many instances, the evaluative design will be part of the program proposal, particularly when the proposal is submitted to a public agency for funding. There may be times, however, when evaluation is planned after a program is well established. Sometimes an evaluation study may be planned to look at only a small portion of the overall program. In these cases, the proposal will be written specifically as a research proposal.

CRITIQUE

When critiquing an evaluation study, internal and external validity must be closely examined. How well the control group was established, whether random assignment was possible, and, if not, how much control was achieved over the action of the independent variable are areas of concern. The internal validity of the study will rest upon these factors.

External validity may be more difficult to assess. Since the program participants are volunteers, it is seldom possible to resolve the external validity issue. The unknown unique characteristics of a volunteer population are always a limiting factor in evaluative studies. Although this problem exists in experimental designs as well, it is not of equal concern, since the major purpose of an experiment is to test theory, not to provide generalizable results. An evaluative study, on the other hand, should provide usable information about the overall effect of the program. Frequently, the results will affect public policy. External validity, therefore, is much more important in this design than it is in experimental designs. Since evaluation studies rarely involve random selection, external validity must be achieved through replication. Bernstein (1976) believes that multiple replications from different populations greatly increase confidence in the results of evaluation studies. From individual studies, however, results must be interpreted with great caution.

REFERENCES

Alwin, D. F., & Sullivan, M. J. (1976). Issues of design and analysis in evaluation research. In I. N. Bernstein (Ed.), *Validity issues in evaluative research*. Beverly Hills, CA: Sage.
Bernstein, I. N. (Ed.). (1976). *Validity issues in evaluative research*. Beverly Hills, CA: Sage.
Borg, W. R., & Gall, M. D. (1983). *Educational research*. New York: Longman.
Boruch, R. F., & Wortman, P. M. (1979). Implications of educational evaluation for evaluation policy. In D. C. Berliner (Ed.), *Review of research in education, 7* (pp. 309-361). Washington, DC: American Educational Research Association.

Cain, G. G., & Hollister, R. G. (1972). The methodology of evaluating social action programs. In P. H. Rossi & W. Williams (Eds.), *Evaluating social programs*. New York: Seminar.

Dela Cruz, F., Jacobs, A., & Wood, M. J. (1986). The educational needs of home health nurses. *Journal of Home Health Nursing, 4*(3), 11-17.

Martinson, I. M., Moldow, D. G., Armstrong, G. D., Henry, W. F., Nesbit, M. E., & Kersey, J. H. (1986). Home care for children dying of cancer. *Research in Nursing and Health, 9*(1), 11-16.

Patton, M. C. (1980). *Qualitative evaluation methods*. Beverly Hills, CA: Sage.

Thurston, N. E., & Dundas, J. B. (1985). Evaluation of an early post partum discharge program. *Canadian Journal of Public Health, 76*(6), 384-387.

12. Methodological Studies: Instrument Development

Merle H. Mishel

Instrumentation, the process of developing a measure of a concept, is of major importance in the structure of a scientific investigation. As discussed in prior chapters, all decisions concerning the structure and conduct of a research study are done to enhance control. The more control evidenced in the methodology of a study, the more confidence the researcher can have in the validity of the findings. The more control that exists over sources of extraneous variables, the fewer alternative explanations can be posited for the study findings.

The strength of study findings is not based solely upon choice of design, sampling decisions, and other means of controlling extraneous variables; it is also due to the amount of control that exists within the indices of the conceptual variables. When the concept of control is applied to measurement, it refers to the ability of instruments to index the concepts with precision, accuracy, and sensitivity. *Precision* refers to the exactness with which the instrument defines the concept, *accuracy* refers to the correctness or truthfulness with which the instrument reports the concept, and *sensitivity* refers to the ability of the instrument to discriminate levels of the concept. The more precise, accurate, and sensitive the instrument is, the more control exists within the study. If the instrument is not very precise, then interpretation of the findings will be confounded. When instruments lack accuracy, the

AUTHOR'S NOTE: *I would like to thank Dr. Carrie Jo Braden for her expert assistance in the discussion of scaling methods, and Dr. Mary R. Lynn for her oustanding skill in editing this chapter.*

hypothesized relationships between variables will appear weaker than if the variables were measured by more accurate tools.

In the arena of instrumentation, the concept of control is translated into the term *measurement error*, the aspect of scores that does not reflect how subjects differ in the amount of the concept being indexed, but reflects scores due to some other influence. Observed scores on a measure equal true score plus error ($x = T + e$). Inaccuracy and imprecision in a measure refer to the amount of measurement error in that instrument. The net effect of measurement error is to lower the degree of correlation. The errors in a set of measures are not correlated, and they make up the portion of the relationship that the set of tests do not have in common. Thus they reduce or attenuate the degree of relation (Guilford, 1936). Because of the attenuation effect, it is necessary to construct instruments with as little measurement error as possible to enhance the strength of the findings.

This chapter will discuss instrument development from the perspective of enhancing control—that is, of decreasing measurement error. Each step in the process of instrument development will be presented in terms of how the activity should be approached to enhance the accuracy, precision, and sensitivity of the final instrument, thereby minimizing measurement error. Measurement error is not an issue to be considered only when reliability and validity testing enter the process of instrument development. Rather, enhancing control by minimizing measurement error permeates each step of the instrument development process. How each step in the instrumentation process relates to the issue of measurement error will be discussed. Published nursing instrumentation studies will be used as examples of specific instrumentation topics, but I take no position concerning the overall quality of any study used as an example.

The field of instrument development is too varied and complex to be presented in a single chapter, thus only major portions of the instrument development process will be discussed here. The reader is referred to other authors for further information throughout the discussion.

Measures in nursing can be used for different purposes, such as discriminating between subjects, predicting the results of some tests, or evaluating change over time. Norm-referenced measures are constructed for the purpose of discriminating between subjects. A specific characteristic is measured in such a way that differences among people who possess differing quantities of that characteristic will be evidenced on the scale. A major feature of this type of measure is variance, that is, the spread of people across a possible range of scores. The goal is to achieve a distribution of scores that resembles a normal curve (Waltz, Strickland, & Lenz, 1984). A predictive index, often referred to as a *criterion-referenced measure,* is constructed for the purpose of determining whether a subject has or has not achieved a predetermined set of target behaviors. The test categorizes individuals into a set of predefined behaviors and can use an external criterion, available either concurrently or prospectively, to determine whether individuals have been classified correctly. A third possible purpose of a nursing instrument is as an evaluation index, for measuring the magnitude of longitudinal change in an individual or a group on a dimension of interest. Such instruments are often used in determining treatment benefit in clinical trials (Kirshner & Guyatt, 1985).

Since the major steps in scale development differ for these different measurement frameworks, it is important that a chapter such as this limit its scope to one framework. The norm-referenced approach, which is the construction of a discriminative index, includes the majority of personality, attitudinal, affective, and cognitive constructs that are developed in nursing. This chapter will focus on methods of test construction that are based on the summative or linear model (Nunnally, 1978). In this model, items are summed to produce a test score. According to Nunnally (1978), there is no general competitor to the linear model. Any measure that is a linear combination of individual responses will fit the principles to be discussed even if the measure has dichotomous items or items scorable on more than two points.

MEASUREMENT ERROR

Zeller and Carmines (1980) present an observation by Hauser in which he proposes that it is inadquate measurement, more than inadequate concepts or hypotheses, that has tormented researchers and that accounts for mediocre explanations from investigators. In order to develop adequate measures, the researcher must understand the nature of the inaccuracy in measurement, so that he or she can avoid it as much as possible.

Errors in measurement are of two types: random error and systematic error. *Random error* refers to random influences that tend to make measurements differ from time to time or cause variations in performance from item to item on a single measure (Nunnally, 1978). Some sources of random error in measures are caused by chance elements with unknown causes, temporary circumstances like fluctuations in memory or mood, momentary states such as irritability or tension, or fluctuating environmental conditions such as heat or noise that effect the object measured or the measuring instrument. Random errors of measurement are never completely eliminated, but efforts can be made to reduce errors as much as possible so that measures are consistent and stable. Random error affects the consistency of measurements, that is, their reliability. Since the reliability of a measure depends upon its degree of consistency and repeatability, as the amount of random error in a measure increases, reliability is reduced (Zeller & Carmines, 1980). An important characteristic of random error is that it causes the measure to appear disorganized, with scores leaning one way at one time and another way at another time. Reliability is determined by the degree of nonrandom error, or true scores, in the instrument (Kerlinger, 1986).

Systematic error refers to systematic influences that distort the scale scores. This source of error has a biasing influence on measurement procedures and influences an instrument's validity. For example, if a thermometer yields exactly the same reading for an individual on 10 different occasions, it is reliable even if it is later discovered that the instrument provided a temperature of 103 degrees fahrenheit for a patient whose actual temperature was 100. Thus the thermometer, as a measure, contains a systematic error, because repeated readings register three degrees higher than they should be. This systematic error clearly compromises the validity of the measurement instrument (Zeller & Carmines, 1980).

Systematic error is due to some characteristic that is regularly tapped by the measure other than that for which the instrument was constructed. If the instrument uniformly stimulates social desirability or encourages always positive or always negative responses, or includes items that measure knowledge skills or abilities irrelevant to the concept being measured, then the instrument contains systematic error (Waltz et al., 1984; Zeller & Carmines, 1980). Other sources of systematic error are not associated with the instrument, but with en-during aspects of the respondent. Such sources include characteristics that are likely to influence responses to the measure in a consistent manner, such as a consistently negative attitude, poor memory, or physical disability. Some of these sources of systemic error can also be implicated in random error. Another major source of systematic error is a situation in which the set of items in a measure index more than the intended theoretical concept, or represent an entirely different concept (Carmines & Zeller, 1980).

Because systemic error has a consistent distorting effect on the scores of an instrument, it is difficult to detect. This source of bias causes a problem with validity because all results obtained with the instrument are contaminated and the accuracy with which the intended concept was indexed is open to question.

To formulate the idea of measurement error, it is necessary to under-stand the role of variance in measurement. Any set of measures has a total variance calculated after determining the mean and standard deviation. The total variance of a measure includes variance due to several causes. The total variance includes true variances, error variance, and systematic variance.

Reliability (r_{tt}) is the proportion of true variance to the total variance of the measure. Reliability also is the proportion of error variance to total variance subtracted from 1.00 (Kerlinger, 1986).

$$r_{tt} = \frac{V_{oo}}{V_t} \qquad r_{tt} = 1 - \frac{V_e}{V_t}$$

As seen in Figure 12.1, in a measure of anxiety the reliability of the measure is 80, because of the total variance, 80% is true variance and 20% is error variance.

Validity is the proportion of total variance of a measure that is com-mon variance, or the variance that the items have in common, that is, that which reflects the concept under measurement. Also included in the total variance of a measure are the random error and systematic variance. As explained earlier, systematic variance must be separated from total variance to determine the validity of the instrument. Valid-ity (r_{xy}) can be viewed as that part of the total variance of a measure that is neither systematic variance nor error variance (Kerlinger, 1986).

$$r_{xy} = \frac{V_t}{V_t} - \frac{V_s}{V_t} - \frac{V_e}{V_t}$$

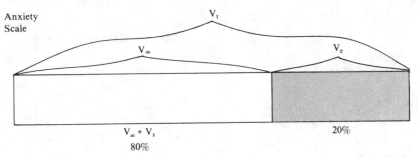

V_t = Total variance
V⁸ = True variance
V_e = Random error variance
V_s = Systematic error variance

Figure 12.1

where V_t = total variance,
 V_s = systematic error variance,
and V_e = random error variance.

Figure 12.2 represents the partitioning of error that must be removed from total variance in order to obtain an estimate of the reliability and validity of an instrument. A paradox exists between random error and systematic error. With systematic error, a measure will appear as more reliable because all items will be similarly affected by the method artifact, yet in such a case the measure will be less valid. With the opposite case, in which items are differentially affected by a chance element—that is, random error—reliability will be relatively lower but the instrument will perform with greater validity. However, since reliability always exceeds validity, although it can be lowered in the case of random error, its mathematical relationship with validity will be preserved. Thus reliability and validity are inextricably bound, and both are influenced by the two types of measurement error (Bohrnstedt, 1970). Consistency among items does not indicate that the tool adequately measures the intended concept, only that whatever it does measure, it measures accurately. An instrument that has low reliability does not represent anything systematically; it cannot represent the concept as intended. Thus for a measure to be valid, it must also be reliable. Reliability is a necessary, but not sufficient, condition for validity (Carmines & Zeller, 1979).

Measurement error, whether random or systematic, is problematic because it tends to attenuate the relationship between variables, thus

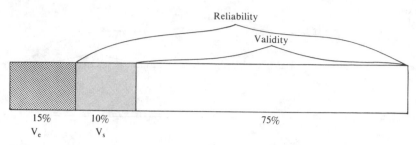

Figure 12.2

weakening the study findings. Both types of error must be controlled to the greatest degree possible. There are well-known and -established methods to test for the presence of random and systematic error in reliability and validity testing procedures. Another approach is to attend to minimizing these error effects in the development of measures. Attention to instrumentation procedures can aid in ensuring that all possible steps are implemented to minimize error and to develop reliable and valid measures.

Concept Clarification

The term *concepts* will be used in this chapter to refer to highly abstract phenomena that can be considered concepts or constructs. The labels *concept* and *construct* will be considered interchangeable. The process of defining the structure of the concept must precede, and be separate from, the development of measurement techniques. The first step in the development of an instrument is to clarify the concept to be measured. This is initiated by developing the theoretical definition and then specifying the variables derived from that definition. Waltz et al. (1984) suggest that in order to formulate a theoretical definition for a concept, investigators must translate their informal working definition into a theoretical definition that is precise, understandable to others, and appropriate for the context in which the term will be used. Walker and Avant (1983) present three basic approaches to clarifying a concept for which an instrument will be developed: analysis, synthesis, and derivation. Each will be discussed, as each is useful in clarifying and defining a concept.

Concept analysis is a useful method for defining a concept when a body of theoretical literature exists. The researcher can carefully review the literature and attend to consistencies and inconsistencies in the use of the concept, the different sources of meaning given to the concept, and subtle differences in how the concept is defined. Before surveying the literature, it is useful to develop a preliminary definition using examples of the concept as it occurs in nursing situations. This helps to indicate the purpose for which the concept is being defined and operationalized.

At the conclusion of a concept analysis based primarily upon a literature review, the researcher should be aware that knowledge of the concept is limited to what is available, tested, or found useful as a definition by others. Literature reviews do not facilitate the emergence of new, creative definitions. The use of concepts from other fields may not be applicable to nursing. Concepts may be defined differently in other areas of the social sciences and may have different dimensions and components than they would have in nursing. Sensitivity to this issue is necessary in order to prevent abstracting definitions from other fields without raising questions about the appropriateness of the definitions when moving concepts from one field to another.

Concept synthesis is a method for developing concepts based on clinical observation; thus it is data based (Walker & Avant, 1983). The process of concept synthesis is useful for building theory and permits the theorist to use clinical experience as a place to begin. Concept synthesis is based upon the exploration of a phenomenon using qualitative methodologies. Data are gathered from clinical interviews and observations and are examined for similarities and differences.

Concept synthesis is a useful means for developing or clarifying a concept in the clinical field. Because the concept emerges from clinical data, there is no question as to its relevance in nursing. In this type of method, there is little question about whether the definition of the concept fits the phenomenon as it exists in nursing. Because this concept emerged from nursing practice and from nursing clinical data, it is grounded in clinical data and thus is a valid description of clinical phenomena (Glaser, 1978).

It is important to note that very few instrumentation studies in nursing have used qualitative methodologies to clarify concepts. It is suggested that qualitative methodologies be used more frequently as a means to generate concepts for measurement within nursing research.

Concept derivation consists of moving a concept from one field of interest to another. In the process of borrowing a concept, the concept must be redefined when moved to a new area of study. Creativity and imagination are necessary in redefining a concept; this is much more than simply assigning a slight modification to it. When a concept is placed into a new field, the definition of it must be innovative, relevant, and meaningful to the new field (Walker & Avant, 1983). When the nursing researcher is considering concept derivation, fields closely related to nursing are preferable and should be those initially explored (Walker & Avant, 1983). Disciplines such as medicine and social work may house relevant concepts, and because these disciplines are closely related to nursing, modification of the concept may be slight or even unnecessary. As there are no rules governing where to search for concepts, the natural and behavioral sciences may also be considered as sources. The main advantage of concept derivation as a strategy is that the researcher need not start from scratch. The use of concepts from other fields often speeds the creative process.

THEORETICAL DEFINITION

After clarifying a concept, the researcher states the theoretical definition and specifies dimensions of the concept. From the literature review, the inductive qualitative study, or from deriving a concept from another field, the researcher is able to identify the dimensions of the concept, which are then specified in the theoretical definition.

Following the theoretical definition, the researcher generates relational statements from the literature or inductive work to provide explanations for the concept and embed it into a theoretical or conceptual framework. Relational statements indicate the association of the concepts. All concepts should be paired with relational statements because this provides a method for testing the construct validity of an instrument.

OPERATIONALIZATION

According to Waltz et al. (1984), the process of operationalizing a concept involves several related steps: (1) developing the theoretical definition, (2) specifying variables derived from the theoretical definition, (3) identifying observable indicators, and (4) developing a means for measuring the indicators.

Movement from the theoretical definition of the concept to the development of the measure happens through the process of operationalization. This is a process of determining and defining how the concept will be measured. In the process of operationalization, the researcher moves from the abstract, which is the concept, to the concrete, the specific observables or items that will index the concept. To operationalize the concept, the researcher specifies the empirical indicators and procedures used to measure it.

The process of moving from a theoretical to an operational definition involves a major component of the validity of the instrument. When the researcher moves from a conceptual variable to an operational variable, the attempt is to structure an operational variable that is isomorphic with the theoretical definition. Isomorphism indicates the degree to which the operational variable is equivalent to the conceptual variable. The term *operational variable* refers to the specific items that will be generated to address the specific aspects of the concept. Operational variables are the actual items developed for the concept. Since concepts are abstract, one never tests them directly, but tests only the operational variables. The definitions of the conceptual variable are used as a guide for selecting the content of the operational variable. The relationship between the conceptual and the operational variable is called the *measurement assumption*.

MEASUREMENT ASSUMPTION

The measurement assumption is the supposition that the operational variable is a clear representation of the conceptual variable. This is the center of the validity issue. Validity testing is an attempt to support the measurement assumption. Validity is concerned with the extent to which one can have confidence in the operational variable as a replica of the conceptual variable. Until a measurement assumption is made, and until the operational variable is defined as an indicator of the conceptual variable, the numbers indexed by the operational variable are relatively meaningless.

One test of the measurement assumption is concerned with the content validity of the instrument. Content validity depends on the extent to which an empirical measurement reflects a specific domain of content (Carmines & Zeller, 1979). Specific steps involved in attaining a content-valid measure will be addressed later in this section. At this point, it should be recognized that items should be developed to reflect isomorphism with the concept and should adequately tap the conceptual domain. Content validity is built into a scale from the initial steps through construction or selection of appropriate items (Anastasi, 1976). Items are designed with the goals of maintaining congruency with the concept definition and of adequately sampling the item universe. When items are inclusive of all dimensions of the conceptual domain, the likelihood of establishing a content-valid measure is enhanced.

A second test of the measurement assumption is concerned with the construct validity of the instrument. Construct validity depends upon the degree to which the empirical measure performs according to theoretical predictions. In order to test the measurement assumption, the conceptual variable must be embedded in theory. A concept in itself has little explanatory value, and becomes meaningful only when placed in a context. For example, a high or low level of anxiety is uninterpretable unless discussed as related to a certain outcome associated with another concept or influenced by another event.

By embedding the conceptual variable into a theoretical statement, a conceptual hypothesis can be formed. This conceptual hypothesis stipulates the relationship between two abstract variables but is never tested directly. Instead, there is indirect testing of the conceptual hypothesis through tests of its corresponding operational hypothesis. In later testing, support for the operational hypothesis provides evidence confirming the measurement assumption. Sustaining the operational hypothesis is evidence that each operational variable is a valid index of its conceptual variable because the operational hypothesis performs as was proposed by the theory, that is, the conceptual hypothesis.

Since the measurement assumption connects the conceptual and operational levels of a theory, the clarity of the theoretical definition will aid in specifying the domain of the operational variable. The specificity with which the domain of the operational variable is defined will mean less slippage when measuring the conceptual variable, thus increasing the probability of supporting the operational hypothesis. Accuracy in determining representative observables to index the concept is an important step in eventual support for the validity of the instrument. This information will be discussed again below, when construct validity is addressed. It is introduced at this point to give the researcher a clear understanding of the importance of defining operational variables so that they correspond with their respective conceptual variables. Ensuring isomorphism between the concept and the operation needs to occur early in the scale development process. Isomorphism should be a definite concern when moving from a theoretical to an operational definition in order to minimize systematic error. This type of error can result when a lack of attention is paid to the domain of observables relevant to the concept and instead observables that index an irrelevant concept are included.

DEVELOPING ITEMS

Concepts vary widely in the extent to which the domain of the observable indicators is either large or small, specifically or loosely defined. If the domain of variables is small, then it will be relatively easy to identify the specific indicators. At a higher level of complexity, typical of concepts that are investigated in nursing research, a large number of observables may be present, making it more difficult to define the concept and to determine which variables do or do not belong in the domain. The more abstract the concept, the greater the number of inferential steps that are necessary to translate observation into meaning (Waltz et al., 1984).

Items should be generated for each dimension of an instrument in such a way that items for each dimension are homogeneous. When all dimensions have item sets, they are combined to constitute the entire instrument. In later reliability testing, each dimension must be analyzed separately because consistency or homogeneity exists within but not across dimensions. Dimensions must, however, evidence a common theme by their intercorrelations.

Attending to the correspondence among items in the process of item development will minimize the degree of random error found in the instrument. When items are generated according to their similarity in thematic content, then each item is less likely to contain irregular characteristics that could stimulate inconsistent responses.

In developing items, the investigator can follow a variety of paths. He or she can use personal judgment concerning items, tap the clinical experience of colleagues, consult the relevant literature, or use more inductive methods, such as interviewing respondents about the concept and how it affects their lives. Regardless of the method used, the investigator must begin with some criteria for inclusion of individual items in the initial pool. It is important to include items that potentially apply to a wide variety of respondents and that are thought to remain stable over short periods of time (Kirshner & Guyatt, 1985). Major criteria for the generation of items include exemplars associated with the conceptual definition and affiliated with other items. These two points are usually considered for inclusion of items, as they address both reliability and validity issues.

A general method for generating items is to review the literature. Most nursing research instruments have been developed through review of published anecdotal studies, case studies, or reports of the experience of specific populations. Statements are identified from this material and converted into items. For examples of the use of this method from the nursing literature, see Baldree, Murphy, and Powers (1982), Jalowiec and Powers (1981), and Cox (1985). Another method for developing items is to use a combination of literature reviews, interviews with consultants or experts in the area, and patient interviews (see Wolf, Putnam, James, & Stiles, 1978). A third method involves selecting items from existing scales. Caution is advised with this method, however, as the investigator must determine whether the conceptual definition used as the basis for the original scale is consistent with the definition of the concept as stated by the present investigator. Items should not be borrowed from existing scales that are based upon different definitions of the concept. A good example of a different approach to the use of items than has been presented is provided by Stevenson (1982). A second example by Hoskins (1981) presents good detail on expanding the original item domain.

The fourth approach to item generation is developing items for a scale from a qualitative investigation of the concept within the target population. This involves interviews with members of the target population to explore the concept. As examples of the concepts emerge, these examples or data bits are categorized according to similar themes. These themes then become the dimensions of the scale and the data bits are reworked into items. Examples of this approach to item development can be found in Mishel (1981) and in Benoliel, McCorkle, and Young (1980). Other examples of the use of qualitative interviews to generate items for a scale are provided by Hymovich (1983) and Cranley (1981).

In the process of developing items for a scale, the researcher must consider whether the scale will index a cognitive process or an attitude/personality variable, because the approach to item development differs based upon the purpose of the scale (Carmines & Zeller, 1979). In order to ensure the content validity of a measure, the approach to the development of items will differ for a cognitive measure compared to an attitudinal or personality measure. According to Lynn (1986), the assessment of content validity should begin at the outset of instrument development. To attend to content validity concerns in the development of a cognitive measure, the researcher should develop the full content domain. For example, if one is attempting to index knowledge about diabetic care, then all of the content concerning diabetic care would need to be identified and categorized. After identifying the content domain, a sample from the different areas of the content would be selected and items generated for each of these sample areas. The researcher need not address every specific area in depth, but should have some items that refer to every major content area of the topic (Lynn, 1986). If instead an attitudinal or personality measure is being developed, then the steps to ensure content validity would differ from those previously identified. The first step in developing an attitude or personality measure is to review the literature, as discussed previously, so that all dimensions and subdimensions of the topic are identified, or to conduct interviews or qualitative work to identify the dimensions that arise inductively. Items are either generated from the literature or translated from the qualitative statements to reflect all of the dimensions. One should try to develop enough items to tap into each dimension fully (Lynn, 1986; Nunnally, 1978). The next step, the same as for cognitive and affective/personality instruments, is to assemble the items into a usable form. This will be discussed in more detail in the next section. The content validity efforts for the developmental stage of an index differ for cognitive and attitudinal/personality instruments (Lynn, 1986).

Developing items to support the content validity of an attitudinal/personality scale is more difficult than doing the same for a cognitive scale. It is easier to specify the domain relevant to a cognitive scale than it is for an affective scale because the cognitive scale will be based on a more specific and concrete domain, whereas the affective scale will be based on a more abstract domain.

ITEM CONSTRUCTION AND RESPONSE CATEGORIES

The term *scale item construction* refers to the way in which the item is structured when it is given to the respondent. In this chapter the focus is on scale items that can be summed to give a total index or measure of the specific concept. The total score is obtained by adding the scores on individual items. Summative scales have a number of advantages over all other methods: (1) They follow from an appealing model; (2) they are relatively easy to construct; (3) they are usually highly reliable; (4) they can be adapted to the measurement of different kinds of attitudes; and (5) they have produced meaningful results in many studies to date.

Considering the nature of the scale items used in summative models, these items can be affected by many problems that contribute to measurement error. Some of the major sources of error in the construction of scale items include the characteristics of the statement itself, such as imperfections, obscurities, and irelevancies. Another problem is that items may be ambiguous in that they refer to two objects at once. Other types of problems stem from items that are obviously redundant, ambiguous, meaningless, or confusing.

Ware, Snyder, McClure, and Jarett (1972) report that Edwards summarized the work of several investigators and developed a list entitled "Informal Criteria for Editing Statements to Be Used in the Construction of Attitude Scales." These informal criteria include 14 separate suggestions:

(1) Avoid statements referring to the past rather than the present.
(2) Avoid factual statements or those that could be interpreted as factual.
(3) Avoid ambiguous statements (those that could be interpreted in more than one way).
(4) Avoid statements irrelevant to the object under study.
(5) Avoid statements likely to be endorsed by almost everyone or almost no one.
(6) Keep language simple, clear, and direct.
(7) Avoid item statements more than 20 words long.
(8) Limit each statement to only one thought.
(9) Avoid statements containing universals (*all, always, none, never*) because they often introduce ambiguity.
(10) Use words such as *only, merely, just,* and others of a similar nature with care and moderation.
(11) Use statements in the form of simple sentences rather than in the form of compound or complex sentences.
(12) Avoid using words that might not be understood by those who are to be given the scale.
(13) Avoid use of double negatives.
(14) Select statements that are believed to cover the entire range of responses concerning the concept of interest.

In the process of developing items, an area of concern is the positive or negative phrasing of items. Nunnally (1978) notes that the purpose of each item on a summary scale is to obtain reliable variance with respect to the concept in question. Most of the items should be moderately positive or moderately negative. Neutral statements should not be used in summative scales. Statements that are very extreme in either direction tend to create less variance than less extreme statements. The pool of items should be about equally divided between positive and negative statements.

Another concern in item construction is the number of items that should be constructed for any scale. Since the major source of error within a test is the sampling of items, the more items in a measure, the less the error (Nunnally, 1978). One can never know for sure how many items should be constructed for a scale until after it is constructed and submitted to item analysis. Item analysis generally shows the number of items that will be needed in order to obtain an acceptable level of reliability. Nunnally (1978) suggests using the Spearman-Brown prophecy formula to estimate how much reliability would be increased if the number of items were increased by any factor. Nunnally (1978) notes that 30 dichotomous items are usually required to obtain an internal consistency reliability of .80. Fewer multipoint items than dichotomous items are required to obtain similar levels of reliability. It is not unusual to find, for example, a coefficient alpha level of .80 for a scale made up of 10 agree-disagree statements rated on a seven-point scale. In order to allow for item analysis to eliminate unsatisfactory items, Nunnally (1978) suggests that 60 items should be constructed initially. Another rule of thumb is that one should generate twice as many items as one would like the final scale to contain. If little is known about the homogeneity of items, then it is wise to be conservative and initially construct more items than necessary.

RESPONSE CATEGORIES

Before subjects can use any scale, steps on the scale must be defined. Definitions of scale steps are referred to as anchors, and there are different types of anchors. Often numbers are used in conjunction with anchors. On percentage scales, subjects rate themselves or others on a continuum ranging from 0 to 100%. The scale is often divided into 10 steps, each corresponding to 10 percentage points, but one can increase the sensitivity of the instrument by employing more finely graded percentage steps.

A second type of anchor frequently used in rating scales is degrees of agreement and disagreement. These scales are easy to work with and are easily understood by subjects. Agreement/disagreement scales are of two types: numerical and graphic. A numerical scale has a set number of steps bounded by statements such as "completely agree" and "completely disagree." In graphic scales, numbers are followed by specific ratings, such as 1 = completely agree, 2 = mostly agree, 3 = slightly agree, 4 = slightly disagree, 5 = mostly disagree, and 6 = completely disagree. The graphic scale is generally considered preferable to the use of numbers alone. Because the graphic scale may remind people of a yardstick or degrees of phenomena, its presence helps to convey the idea of a rating continuum. Also, with the use of the graphic scale there are fewer clerical errors in recording ratings.

Attitudes constitute the third type of anchor for rating scales. Scales often are anchored by two terms, such as valuable-worthless, or effective-ineffective. Attitude scales using bipolar adjective pairs as anchors are easily constructed and can be applied to many types of attitudinal objects. A rating scale using bipolar adjective pairs as anchors is called a *semantic differential*, which is a type of scaling. The semantic differential will be discussed in the section on scaling.

Another concern in constructing items is the number of scale steps. There is always an advantage to using more rather than fewer steps. This is demonstrated by numerous studies showing that the reliability of a scale is a monotonically increasing function of the number of steps (Nunnally, 1978). As the number of scale steps increases from 2 up through 20, the increase in reliability is very rapid at first. It tends to level off at about 7, and after about 8 steps, there is little reliability by increasing the number of steps. Nunnally (1978) notes that as the number of scale points increases, error variance increases, but at the same time the true score increases at an even more rapid rate.

The question of the number of steps in a rating scale is very important if one is dealing with only one item, but it is less important if scores are summed over a number of items. When only one item is used to measure a concept (a practice that is not recommended) there should be at least 10 steps. If there are a limited number of items on the scale, the reliability of a dichotomous scale could be greatly increased by increasing the number of scale steps on the individual scales. On the other hand, when there are more than 20 items in a summated scale, the reliability is not greatly increased by the addition of scale steps to the individual scales. Nunnally (1978) recommends that in nearly all instances it is safer to have at least 5 or 6 steps than it is to have a dichotomous scale. Seldom are there practical advantages to having only two steps.

Another issue regarding the number of steps on rating scales concerns whether an even or an odd number of steps is preferable. Some argue for an odd number of steps to allow for a middle or neutral step, because they believe that subjects are more comfortable making decisions if a neutral reaction is an option. On the other hand, some feel that having a neutral step induces response styles, with some subjects tending to use the neutral step more often than others. Nunnally (1978) concludes that the issue of whether to have a neutral step is not very important, particularly if scores are summed over a number of items.

To emphasize what was stated earlier, it is more important to do everything possible to prevent measurement error from occurring than to try to assess the effects of measurement error after it has occurred. In the area of item construction, measurement error can be reduced by writing items clearly, by making test instructions easily understood, by adhering closely to the prescribed condition for administering an instrument, and by increasing the length of the measure. Measurement error caused by subjectivity in scoring can be reduced when the rules for scoring are as explicit as possible.

SCALING

There are a number of methods available for distinguishing among objects or individuals in terms of the degree to which they possess a given characteristic. Each of these methods involves placing the person or object being rated at some point along a continuum or into one of an ordered series of categories, and attaching a numerical value to that point or category. Scale types discussed here include differential, summated, and cumulative scales, as well as scales that are modifications of these basic forms. Because the object of scaling is to quantify accurately the most comprehensive, complete information for the least overall cost and with the least amount of measurement error, specific

scale types are discussed in terms of their advantages and disadvantages.

In an effort to reduce error involved in rating others on the basis of
observed behavior or responses to open-ended questions, standardized questionnaires have been developed based on expression of agreement or disagreement with a number of statements relevant to the
dimension(s) of interest. In the process of standardizing the questionnaire, the investigator establishes a basis of interpreting agree-
ment/disagreement response-assigned scores as indicating positions
on the dimension. The separate items on such a scale are not of interest in themselves. Rather, researcher interest is in each individual's
total score or in subscores that result from combinations of individual
responses to various item subsets. The way a particular type of scale
discriminates among individuals depends on how the scale is constructed and on the method of scoring. In the following discussion,
the major types of scales used in nursing research will be presented.
For further information on scale construction and scoring, see Kerlinger (1986).

Differential Scales

A differential scale consists of a number of ranked items, whereby
the items themselves form a gradation. The individual will likely agree
with only one or two items corresponding to the individual's position
on the dimension being measured and will likely disagree with items
at all other points on the dimension.

The Thurstone scale is the most common example of the differential
scale type. Establishing the order of the items to approximate equal
intervals is one of the major tasks in construction of a Thurstone scale.
The various methods of providing accurate judgments of scale position include the method of paired comparisons (Thurstone, 1927, 1928),
the method of equal-appearing intervals (Thurstone, 1929; Thurstone
& Chave, 1929), and the method of successive intervals, which is most
commonly selected.

This scale type allows for comparisons of changes in an individual's
position on the dimension or for comparisons across individuals of differences relative to the dimension. Investigations have demonstrated
that the procedure seeking to create equal-appearing intervals does provide an interval scale. The resulting data can be appropriately analyzed
with parametric statistics.

Disadvantages include the amount of work and time necessary for securing the statements and judgments. Scale construction costs are significant. Item selection based on judged agreement tends to result in the elimination of items that less clearly manifest the dimension. Items included in the scale can be considered transparent, with subjects easily able to discern the "socially acceptable" response pattern. Such scales may be more open to social desirability bias. Issues can also be raised regarding the scoring procedure. Because an individual's score is the mean (or median) of scale values assigned to items checked, different response patterns can be expressed by the same score. Two individuals could be rated as having the same degree of prejudice even though one subject checked two moderately "anti" items and the other checked four items representing two "anti" positions and two "pro" positions. In general, the greatest disadvantage of this type of scale is its decreased reliability in comparison with some other types of scales due to reliance on choice between dichotomous responses for each item. The subject either agrees or disagrees with a given item and is not able to indicate more subtle responses that lie between the two extremes (Title & Hill, 1967).

Summative Scales

Like differential scales, the summative scale offers the subject a set of items and requests a response to the items. Items that reflect divergent positions on the dimension are selected, and neutral or moderate (midline) and very extreme aspects of the dimension are omitted. Subjects respond to each item rather than only to those with which they agree. Each response is assigned a numerical score; it is part of instrument development to decide whether favorable or unfavorable responses will be scored positively. The sum of scores of the individual's responses to all items yields the total score and is interpreted as the subject's position relative to the measured dimensions.

The most common type of summative scale is the Likert-type scale. This is the scale type most often selected as the scaling method for measurement of concepts of interest to nurses. In a Likert-type scale, subjects respond to each item in terms of several degrees of agreement or disagreement. Five categories of response are common and are often stated as (1) strongly agree, (2) agree, (3) undecided, (4) disagree, and (5) strongly disagree.

The Likert-type scale is "subject centered" (Torgerson, 1958), having as its purpose the scaling of respondents, not the scaling of the dimension. Any item found empirically to be consistent with the total score can be included. The Likert-type scale is practical in terms of construction costs. The assumptions relative to scoring the Likert-type scale are also lenient relative to measurement error. Because each item may contain considerable measurement error, no single item in summative scales is considered separately. Rather, each item is monotonically related to the underlying dimension continuum. This assumption does not imply that each item has exactly the same level of contribution to the dimension. It states only that the sum of the items is expected to contain all the important information relative to a single common factor (McIver & Carmines, 1978). Because the five-point response format for each item allows more response alternatives, the reliability of the Likert-type scale is likely to be greater than that of a Thurstone scale having the same number of items. This range of responses also provides more precise information about the individual's position on the dimension as referred to by the given item.

Disadvantages of the Likert-type scale include the potential for introduction of response set bias due to inclusion of positively worded statements versus negatively worded statements. The inclusion of an approximately equal number of negatively worded and positively worded items partially controls for response set bias.

As in the Thurstone scale, the total score of the Likert-type scale can represent diverse response patterns. The safeguard against having a meaningless total score is careful item analysis, ensuring that only items that discriminate between high and low scorers are retained. In addition, a rigorous testing schedule is required to determine (1) whether responses remain stable over time, (2) if alternative tests are available, whether individuals receive the same score on different forms, and (3) whether different individuals achieving the same score in different ways react in the same way to particular stimuli, problems, and so on, with the ultimate question being concerned with estimating scale validity. The severest criticism of Likert-type scales has been the fact that such scales can claim to provide only ordinal-level measurement. There has been much debate over the kind of statistical analysis that is appropriate for data provided through Likert-type scales (Armstrong, 1981; Burke, 1953; Labovitz, 1967; Nagel, 1974; Stevens, 1951).

Cumulative Scales

Cumulative scales, like differential and summative scales, offer the respondent a series of items requiring an agreement or disagreement response. But, unlike the other scales, cumulative scales contain items that are related in an incremental fashion. Ideally, a subject replying favorably to item 2 would also reply favorably to item 1; one who replies favorably to item 3 would also reply favorably to items 1 and 2. The individual's score is computed by counting the number of items answered favorably. The total score places the person on the scale of favorable-unfavorable attitude provided by the relationship of items to one another. Items can appear on the scale in order of favorableness or can be randomly arranged.

The Guttman scale is an example of a cumulative scale that also attempts to determine the unidimensionality of the scale. The Guttman technique, although providing a method for determining the unidimensionality of an item set, provides little guidance for selecting items that are likely to form a scale. The Guttman-type scale is useful when examining small changes or shifts in the dimension of interest. It has the potential to serve as a criterion-referenced instrument if items are selected relative to a set of predictable target behaviors.

Disadvantages of the Guttman scale include high costs of construction due to difficulty in initially selecting items likely to be scalable, and to the fact that items may be scalable for one population but not for another. Scalability must be checked prior to use with a population other than that used in initial development. Scalogram analysis is usually performed on one or more samples of 100, with no certainty that a usable scale will emerge from the testing.

Other Scale Types

The scale discrimination technique advocated by Edwards and Kilpatrick (1948) borrows aspects of the construction of Thurstone's equal-appearing intervals, Likert's summated scales, and Guttman's scale analysis to develop a set of items that meet the requirements of unidimensional scales, possess equal-appearing intervals, and measure intensity. Although providing a scale with desired qualities of unidimensionality, interval-level measurement, and measurement of intensity, the construction procedure is very costly. And, in the Guttman procedure for scaling, there is no certainty that a usable scale will emerge from the testing.

The semantic differential scale developed by Osgood, Suci, and Tannenbaum (1957) provides another method for measuring the meaning of an object to an individual. The semantic differential does not place individuals on an underlying scale representing some dimension of a concept; it instead provides a method for measuring the similarity or difference in how respondents view the dimension. Responses to scale subgroups can be summed to yield scores interpreted as the individual's position on three underlying dimensions of attitude: evaluation, potency, and activity. The actual analysis of a semantic differential scale includes a variety of measures that exceed the scope of this chapter. For an excellent discussion of these analyses, see Kerlinger (1986).

The visual analog scale is a type of graphic rating scale that can be used to bypass language limitations. It typically consists of a 100 mm horizontal or vertical line anchored at each end with a brief verbal description of a feeling (Bond & Lader, 1974), mood (Aitkin & Zealley, 1970), or the like to be evaluated relative to the dimension being evaluated. This scale has been used most frequently to measure pain (Huskisson, 1974). The anchored endpoints represent opposing positions. The subject places a mark on the line at the point best representing response to the item. Construction benefits of the visual analog scale are comparable to those discussed for summated scales. The visual analog scale provides a means for evaluating fine changes, and it has been shown to provide increased sensitivity and decreased divergent interpretations (Maxwell, 1978).

PRETESTING

Before an instrument is used in a structured investigation, pretesting of the instrument should occur in order to address many early questions in instrument development. Fox and Ventura (1983) note that pretesting is not frequently done and present two reasons this important step is often bypassed in the process of instrument development. The first relates to the organization of academic disciplines, in which there is a high demand placed upon the individual to produce findings from research investigations and publish as soon as possible. The time and effort that pretesting entails is therefore not encouraged, often at the expense of quality results. The second reason focuses upon the teacher/student relationship. Since pretesting is infrequently conducted, many mentoring relationships do not include role modeling regarding pretesting of instruments. Although Fox and Ventura (1983) note that pretesting can cover an assortment of activities that may include informal opinions from colleagues or more formal testing using small samples that resemble the population of interest, pretesting most correctly refers to formal testing with representative samples of persons.

Pretesting involves determining the feasibility of using a given instrument in a formal study. It provides an opportunity to try out the technique or the instructions that will be used with an instrument, especially if it has never been used with a specific population. Pretesting also allows the researcher an opportunity to simulate the conditions of the study and get some direct experience with what will happen. Through subsequent pretesting, data can be obtained from item analysis. Nunnally (1978) notes that the pretest population should be similar to the group with which the final instrument will be used. It is important that the data for item analysis be obtained under conditions very similar to those in which the final scale will be used. Consistency should be maintained between the type of instructions used in the pretest and those used with the final instrument.

Wolf et al. (1978) provide a fine example of the use of multiple field trials in the development of an instrument. Three pretests or field trials were conducted; each had a specific focus for instrument development. In the first pretest, items were presented to about 50 subjects similar to the target population. The subjects were asked to give feedback about the items in the scale in terms of the appropriateness and clarity of item wording. Based upon this information, some of the items were reworded. A second pretest was aimed at item analysis. Similar subjects were asked to complete the initial form of the scale. Two types of item analysis resulted from the data from the pretest, which then functioned to modify the scale. In the third pretest, the revised form of the scale was administered to about 50 subjects who were the target population of a larger study. The data from the third pretest was again used for item analysis and for validity testing. This example demonstrates the continual evolvement in instrumentation that occurs as a result of well-planned pretests.

A pretest can be used to determine the base rate of the concept being measured. Derogatis and Spencer (1984) note that a problem exists with what they call "base rates," or the predictive value of a measuring instrument when the prevalence rates of the concept are particularly low. As the base rate or the occurrence of the concept becomes markedly low—that is, it pertains to less than 10% of the population—increasingly high sensitivity in the measuring instrument is required to achieve useful measurement. One advantage of pretesting is that it allows the researcher, if using a representative population, to get some index of the prevalence of the concept before further work is put into developing an instrument for a concept that may have a very low level of existence.

Fox and Ventura (1983) present a list of suggestions for conducting a pretest. Some of these are as follows: Allow sufficient time before the actual study to analyze the data and make changes in data collection procedures as necesssary; do not start the study until the pretest results have been analyzed for reliability and validity; try out multiple methods of data collection in order to decide upon a method; if major modifications must be made due to the results of the pretest, then conduct another pretest before a major study is undertaken; conduct several phases of the pretest, as discussed in the example by Wolf et al. (1978); after the pretest, ask subjects to identify any problems they had completing the questionnaire as well as any suggestions they might have for improving the questions; perform item analysis on the pretest data; pretest the questionnaire items on as many types of people as available who will be in the eventual study group; use a sample size of 10 or 20 for a pretest, unless the instrument is complex or the sample is heterogeneous, in which case use a larger sample.

Although the subjects in the pretest are similar to the subjects who will use the final scale, they need not be exact representatives of the test population. Since the test will be used with many types of subjects, it is important that, in the pretest, the sample group be highly representative of all the different groups with which the test will eventually be used. Although Fox and Ventura (1983) say that a pretest may have a small sample, Nunnally (1978) suggests that the scale should initially be administered to 10 times as many subjects as there are items. Although Nunnally supports using a large sample for gathering data for item analysis, it is rarely possible to obtain such a large population in studies using clinical samples. Published instrumentation articles in the nursing research literature generally involve a smaller sample size than proposed. For examples of the use of pretests in nursing, see Cox (1985) and Stevenson (1982).

ITEM ANALYSIS

Item analysis is a procedure to estimate the reliability and determine the validity of a test by separately evaluating each item of the instrument to ascertain whether or not that item discriminates in the same way the overall test is intended to discriminate, and whether the item is of appropriate difficulty (Isaac & Michael, 1974). The content of the final instrument must depend on how the item performs in the setting in which the index will ultimately be used. Therefore, performance criterion must be established so that items that do not contribute to or actually detract from the total instrument can be detected and eliminated in order to strengthen the reliability and validity of the measure. Discriminative criteria are usually structured around two major performance criteria: (1) the discriminability of the item and (2) the accuracy/precision of the item. Discriminability of the item can be tested using three procedures: (1) the discrimination index, (2) split-group response, and (3) two-group response (Isaac & Michael, 1974; Waltz et al., 1984). These three methods assess an item's ability to discriminate, that is, to determine whether the performance of a given item is a good predictor of the performance of the overall measure.

In the discrimination index, to determine the discrimination or D value for a given item, Waltz et al. (1984) provide the following instructions: (1) Rank all subjects' performance on the measure by using total scores from high to low; (2) identify those individuals who ranked in the upper third; (3) identify those individuals who ranked in the lower third; (4) place the remaining scores aside; (5) determine the proportion of respondents in the upper third who answered the item correctly (Pu); (6) determine the proportion of respondents in the lower third who answered the item correctly (Pl); (7) calculate D, D = Pu − Pl; (8) repeat steps 5 through 7 for each item on the measure. D ranges from −1.00 to +1.00. It is desirable to obtain D values greater than +0.20. A positive D value is what is sought, and this indicates that the item discriminates in the same manner as the total test, which means that those who score high on the total test tend to respond the same way on the item. Conversely, those who socre low on the item also tend to score low on the total test. Waltz et al. (1984) state that a negative D value indicates that the item does not discriminate like the total test, and that respondents who score low on the total test tend to get the item correct and vice versa. Thus a negative D value indicates that the item is not a good discriminator and possibly should be removed from the scale.

The split-group response is another procedure that functions like the discrimination index to identify how well an item discriminates relative to the way that the overall test is intended to discriminate. In the split-group response method, subjects are ranked according to the upper and lower half following Steps 1 through 4 for determining D. Following this, a fourfold table is constructed based on two pairs of categories. The first pair is the category high scores versus the low scores, depending on how the ranks are divided. In the next step, the chi-square value of the resulting proportion is calculated using the standard shortcut formula for the chi-square. If the chi-square is significant, it can be concluded that a significant difference has been found in the proportion of high- and low-scoring subjects who gave correct answers. Items that meet this criterion should be retained and items that fail to meet it should be discarded or modified to increase their discriminability.

The third method, the two-group response, is a technique used to discriminate between the responses of two groups given a series of items. For example, one might want to discriminate between medical patients and surgical patients in terms of a specific concept. In this procedure, a contingency table is established, with the two groups being compared constituting the rows and the item response options the columns. For each item, the frequency of each item response by group members is determined and subjected to a chi-square test. If the chi-square value is significant, then it can be concluded that one group responded to the item differently than the other group. If the response is in the direction expected, then the item would be discriminating as expected and would be retained. If the two groups fail to show any difference on an item, then the item would not be discriminating and would either be removed from the scale or modified and retested to increase its discriminatory power (Isaac & Michael, 1974).

Another method for assessing the performance of an item is to determine its accuracy or precision. This method involves determining the item-total correlations, using the Pearson product-moment correlation (biserial correlations for dichotomous items) to derive an indication of how strongly an item reflects the total scale. Since the goal of norm-referenced or discriminative scales is to be able to discriminate between people according to the specific concept under investigation, item reduction methods that delete items not stressing the same theme function to improve the power of the scale to discriminate between two people on the specific variable. The precision of the index will increase based upon the strength with which each individual item relates to the total scale.

In item analysis with item-total correlations, the first step is to determine the actual correlations. Then items are ordered based on the correlations, with the item with the highest correlation ranked first. Approximately 30 items is a common instrument length. The top 30 items, based on the item-total correlations, are selected to constitute the instrument. Even if all or almost all of the items in the original pool have high item-total correlations, they may or may not end up in the final instrument depending on the reliability of the instrument.

Generally, the items having the highest item-total correlation are selected. Items with low item-total correlation are deleted. If the internal consistency of the scale is computed at this time, it can be determined whether adding items or deleting items raises or lowers the level of reliability. If reliability is sufficiently high with the items having the highest item-total correlation, then there is little to be gained by adding more items.

Nunnally (1978) advises that when one has multipoint items it is wise to compute the internal consistency for the 10 items having the highest correlations with total scores, and if reliability is not high enough, to add several items until the desired reliability is obtained. Nunnally (1978) presents several reasons this method may fail to produce a homogeneous test. One of the most common is that the collection of items is factorially complex. Some items correlate strongly within themselves, but have low correlations with other items, thereby preventing a homogeneous scale from being formed. If the researcher has hypothesized a number of factors, each of which relates to different attributes of the concept, and there are sufficient subjects with which to do so (n = 5-10 subjects per item), he or she should proceed to factor analyze the item pool initially, rather than attempt the construction of a homogeneous scale. When a factor analysis is planned, the sample should be carefully selected to be representative of the kind of population to which the investigator will generalize the findings, and must be large enough to give stable correlation coefficients.

Carmines and Zeller (1979) note that factor analysis is explicitly designed to address the situation in which the items in the scale are not unidimensional. This implies that the items as a group do not measure a single phenomenon but rather measure more than one phenomenon or aspects of a phenomenon. Factor analysis is a statistical method used to discover clusters of interrelated variables. When an instrument addresses several phenomena or aspects of a phenomenon, items tend to fall in clusters or factors. The items composing a factor are more highly correlated with each other than were the other items. Factor analysis is introduced here to explain that when factors have been incorporated into the construction of a scale, factor analysis should precede investigation of item-total correlations. After factor analysis has been computed, item-total correlations can then be meaningfully computed for each of the factors. Items that do not load heavily on a factor can be deleted. *Loading* refers to the extent to which each item is correlated with every other item on the factor. The higher the item loads on the factor, the more the particular item contributes to that factor. This is an alternative way to look at item-total correlations. Items that load heavily on a factor would then be retained and items with weak loadings on the factor would be deleted. For more information on traditional factor loadings considered appropriate during factor analysis, the reader is referred to texts on the topic. Some examples of the use of factor analysis as a basis for item deletion can be found in the work of Mishel (1981, 1983). Other examples of the use of criteria for item-total correlations can be found in the work of Stevenson (1982), Cox (1958), and Cranley (1981).

RELIABILITY

Reliability refers to the degree of consistency and repeatability of the scores on an instrument. A measure that is unreliable shows scores that are variable and fluctuating. Reliability is equal to the observed variance that is not random or fluctuating, but is repeatable or true. Systematic error is not an issue in reliability because, since it is not random, it does not reduce consistency and repeatability. The culprit in reliability is random error. When random error is low, reliability is high. The reliability coefficient is the portion of test variance that is true or nonrandom variance. If, for example, a reliability coefficient is .70, then 70% of the variance in scores is due to variation in true differences between the subjects on the concept under measurement. The remaining 30% of the variance is due to inaccuracy in the measurement (Isaac & Michael, 1974).

Types of Reliability

Test-Retest

The test-retest method is appropriate for determining the reliability of a measure when the concept being tested is thought to be relatively stable over the time period in which the testing will occur. Test-retest procedures are often used to determine the reliability of affective measures and attitudes. Since cognitive measures may change rapidly, this procedure is not usually used for such an instrument. With the test-retest procedure, the investigator is concerned with the consistency of measurement in the same group of subjects from Time 1 to Time 2. Waltz et al. (1984) present the following three-step procedure to estimate test-retest reliability for a specific measure: (1) Under standardized conditions, give the measure to a single group of subjects who represent the group for which the measure was developed. (2) Give the test again, two weeks later, to the same group of people under the same conditions (the time between tests may vary slightly). It is important to note whether any new activities occur between the first and second administration that may effect the consistency of the concept being measured. (3) Determine the extent to which the two sets of scores are correlated. If the data are considered interval level, Pearson product-moment correlation is customarily used as the estimate of reliability; if the data are at a nominal or ordinal level, a nonparametric measure of association is used. The reliability coefficient from the test-retest procedure is called the *coefficient of stability* because it measures the extent to which subjects perform at the same level on two separate occasions. The higher the coefficient of stability, the more stable the measuring device is assumed to be. For examples of the use of this method in nursing research, see Baldree et al. (1982), Jalowiec and Powers (1981), Hoskins (1981), and Norbeck, Lindsey, and Carrieri (1981).

Although test-retest may be an appealing procedure, it is not without serious problems. Zeller and Carmines (1980) note that researchers are often able to obtain a measure of a phenomenon at a single point in time, but it can be very expensive and impractical to obtain measures at various points in time. Even if test-retest correlations can be accomplished, their interpretation is often ambiguous. A low test-retest corelation may not indicate that reliability is low, but instead indicate that the concept itself has changed. The longer the time interval between measures, the more likely it is that the concept has changed.

Knapp (1985) discusses some of the errors that frequently occur in nursing research concerning test-retest reliability. Test-retest reliability is meant to provide some evidence over a brief period of time regarding the short-term consistency of measures yielded by a particular test. It is not usually concerned with long-term consistency of the concept being measured. Often the word *stability* is associated with reliability studies carried out over a brief period of time in which the investigator is concerned with the consistency of the concept instead of with the consistency of the scores. It is important to distinguish between a test-retest reliability study and study of a particular concept. If scores change over the time period selected, presuming the interval between administration was appropriately selected for the concept studied, then the instrument is assessed as not being stable (reliable) rather than the concept being noted as changed in those studied. Concept changes cannot reliably be identified using an unreliable instrument.

If the construct being measured is a trait, this will present different problems than if the concept is defined as a state. Traits are considered enduring, whereas states—emotions such as anxiety or depression—may be considered transitory. In order to use test-retest methods, the concept being measured should be conceptualized as a trait behavior and the level of the concept should not change over time. If an attitude or belief system is being measured, this is assumed to be relatively stable unless some unusual environmental event occurs, and thus should remain stable over time. If the behavior exists in a transition state, test-retest methods can be utilized if an appropriate interval can be determined. Use of test-retest methods is based on the understanding that the ability of the instrument to produce the same score is being tested, not the ability of the concept to remain stable or fluctuate.

A second problem with the test-retest method is that it can lead to deflated reliability estimates due to reactivity. Reactivity is what happens when measuring a phenomenon induces change in the phenomenon itself. If a person's belief concerning a concept is measured at Time 1, he or she may become sensitized, and may demonstrate a change at Time 2.

If the test-retest correlation is low, the alternate form correlation will be even lower. If the test does not correlate with itself when given on two separate occasions, then it is less likely to correlate with another test measuring the same concept. Examples of the use of the test-retest method can be found in Hoskins (1981) and Norbeck et al. (1981).

Equivalence

The major method for achieving equivalence of a test involves using two different forms of an instrument to measure the same concept. In this form of reliability, one is attempting to determine whether there will be consistent performance on two different forms of a measure by the same subjects during one specific testing period. The two different measures are considered alternative or parallel forms if they have some of the following characteristics: They were constructed using the same objective procedures and based upon the same conceptual definition, they have approximately equal means, they correlate about equally with any third variable, and they have equal standard deviations (Waltz et al., 1984). To conduct the alternate forms method, both instruments are given to the subjects on the same measurement occasion. The extent to which the two sets of scores are correlated is determined using an appropriate statistic for the level of measurement in both measures. If the measures correlate highly, then they are seen as equivalent. If the correlation is above .80, this indicates that the forms may be used interchangeably. For examples of the use of alternate forms as a measure of reliability in nursing research, see Hoskins (1981, 1983).

Internal Consistency

The two methods subsumed under internal consistency are the most basic and popular ways of estimating reliability. This method for assessing reliability focuses on multiple indicators of a concept measured at a similar point in time. Each indicator, usually an item, is considered a separate but equal measure of the underlying concept. The early measure of internal consistency focused on split-half methods. In these methods the total number of items were divided into two halves and the correlation between the two halves provided an estimate of the reliability of all of the items. The problem with this method is that the point at which each split occurs will produce a different correlation between the halves. This leads to differences in reliability estimates. Other problems with this method are that it applies mostly to cognitive measures, assumes that item content is evenly spread, and is not useful when the instrument is not fully completed by some respondents.

In response to some of the problems in estimating reliability by the use of the split-half method, other methods have been developed that do not require the splitting or repeating of items, but still provide a measure of internal consistency. Of all of the methods to determine internal consistency, the method that is most popular and most generally applicable is Cronbach's coefficient alpha. Coefficient alpha is equal to the average of all possible split-half correlations for composite scales that are N items long (Zeller & Carmines, 1980). Alpha takes scores varying between 0 and +1, taking these extremes when the item correlations can be equal to 0 in unity or be perfect and equal to 1 (Zeller & Carmines, 1980). Generally, as the number of items on a scale increases, the average correlation among the items increases and alpha takes on a larger value. The criterion level for coefficient alpha with a new scale has been suggested to be at about .70 or above, and for a mature scale .80 or above (Nunnally, 1978).

When considering intercorrelations between items in a scale, it is important that the correlations be high enough to index similarity between the items and yet not be so high that they index redundancy. Interitem correlations should average between .30 and .70. Correlations above .70 imply redundancy and items at that point can be deleted (Gordon, 1968).

To measure internal consistency, two different estimates are used. Cronbach's alpha is applicable to scales with multiple responses, and the Kuder-Richardson 20 is applicable to cognitive scales with dichotomous items. KR-20 is the most useful reliability coefficient for dichotomous items because it makes no special assumptions regarding the distribution of items. Alpha measures the extent to which performance of any one item on an instrument is a good indicator of performance of any other item on the same instrument. Thus the addition of items to an instrument, if it does not result in a reduction in the average interitem correlation, will increase reliability.

A number of characteristics of the measurement situation can affect the alpha value that is obtained. Alpha is a function of test length; the longer the test, the higher the level of alpha. The second characteristic of coefficient alpha is that it increases with the spread of variance of scores. Perhaps the most important characteristic to remember concerning coefficient alpha is that alpha equals reliability only if the items are strictly parallel. Otherwise the value of alpha merely sets a lower bound on the reliability; that is, the reliability of the scale cannot be less than the value noted for alpha. Alpha does not provide a very good estimate of reliability when the items making up the scale are heterogeneous in their relationship to each other or when their number is small. In each of these conditions, alpha will be smaller than the true internal consistency of the scale. When interitem correlations are low, the value given by alpha understates the true reliability. Zeller and Carmines (1980) note that there are two conditions under which alpha may not provide a good estimate of reliability: (1) if the items measure a single concept unequally or (2) if the items measure more than one concept equally or unequally.

Although there are some limits to the conditions under which alpha can provide a good estimate of reliability, there are still many points in favor of using this measure of internal consistency. Kirshner and Guyatt (1985) note that coefficient alpha provides a good estimate of measurement error attributable to inappropriate or inadequate sampling of content domain. It is important to be able to determine what sources of error have been addressed by a specific reliability coefficient. Coefficient alpha is excellent for addressing sources of error due to inappropriate or inadequate sampling of items, which is the major source of error within a test. Nunnally (1978) goes further, noting that all of the types of errors that occur within a test can easily be handled by this measure of internal consistency. The general consensus is that coefficient alpha provides a good, albeit occasionally conservative, estimate of reliability in most situations.

It has also been shown that reliability estimates based on internal consistency also consider sources of error that are not, strictly speaking, due to the sampling of items but to the sampling of situational factors that accompany the administration of items. Many of these sampling decisions, noted by Isaac and Michael (1974), that can be potential sources of error are adequately handled by coefficient alpha. Coefficient alpha is frequently used as an estimate of reliability in nursing research. For examples of its use, see Hinshaw and Atwood (1982), Mishel (1983), and Murphy, Powers, and Jalowiec (1985).

Some conditions limit the usefulness of alpha as a reliability estimate. Alpha may underestimate the "true" reliability of an instrument composed of separate factors or subscales because there will be more consistency within these factors or subscales than when they are considered as a whole instrument. In such cases, reliability estimates should be obtained for each subscale as well as for the total scale.

When analyzing the reliability of scales that contain more than one dimension, the coefficients omega and theta represent the internal consistency of the items within each subscale. Coefficient theta and coefficient omega, the types of reliability coefficients used in factor analysis, have some important differences. Each coefficient is based on a different factor-analytic model. Theta is used with the principal components model, whereas omega is based on the common factor analysis model. Theta can be understood most simply as being a special case of coefficient alpha. Although theta and alpha are grounded in different factor analysis models, there are also some similarities between them. If the items constituting a scale are parallel measures, then all three coefficients—alpha, theta, and omega—should be equal to one another and will equal the reliability of the scale. If the items are not parallel, omega will have the highest value, followed by theta and finally by alpha. Alpha is the lower limit for the reliability of a multi-item scale. Of all these three internal consistency coefficients, omega provides the highest estimate of reliability, that is, the closest to the true reliability of the instrument (Carmines & Zeller, 1979). There are assumptions about theta and omega that should be considered preceding their use. For information on these assumptions, the reader is referred to texts on factor analysis.

VALIDITY

Validity refers to the ability of an instrument to measure exactly what it is supposed to measure and nothing else. In order to determine the validity of an instrument, the researcher should consider the major reasons it was developed or the major functions it serves. Instruments serve three major functions: (1) to represent the universe of content related to a specific concept, (2) to establish a relationship with a particular variable, and (3) to measure attitudinal, affective behavior or cognitive variables (Nunnally, 1978). There are three types of validity; each represents a response to one of the three functions of an instrument: (1) Content validity relates to the representation of a specific universe of content, (2) criterion-related validity relates to establishing a relationship with a particular variable, and (3) construct validity relates to measurement of specific psychological variables.

A second approach to conceptualizing validity testing is in terms of two types of evidence: internal association and external association (Zeller & Carmines, 1980). *Internal association* refers to the pattern of interrelationships among the indicators designed to measure the concept. This can encompass the methods of determining content validity. *External association* refers to the pattern of relationships between items designed to measure a concept and other variables. External association can encompass criterion-related and construct validity methods.

Content Validity

The term *content validity* refers to an estimation of the adequacy with which a specific domain of content is sampled. It refers to the content representativeness of the concept; that is, the completeness with which items cover the important areas of the domain they are attempting to represent. To the degree that the items reflect the full domain of content, they can be said to be content valid.

Content validity has been criticized in the instrumentation literature due to the lack of agreed-upon criteria for establishing whether a measure has obtained content validity. Nunnally (1978) had noted that "inevitably content validity rests mainly on appeals to reason regarding the adequacy with which important content has been sampled and on the adequacy in which the content has been cast in the form of test items."

Recent work has occurred in nursing that attempts to quantify the content validity process (see Lynn, 1986). Earlier in this chapter, the first step in assessing content validity was discussed for item development for either a cognitive or an affective/personality instrument. The second stage in assessing content validity is the judgment/quantification stage, which involves selecting experts to evaluate the content validity of each item and of the total scale (Lynn, 1986).

Lynn (1986) identifies the process for quantifying content validity as determining the number of experts needed to evaluate the items and the proportion who must agree in order for content validity to be established. It is recommended that specific guidelines be applied for the selection of experts. A minimum of three is recommended in order to obtain statistically justifiable results. For more than three available judges, Lynn provides a table for determining the proportion of experts who must agree in order to establish content validity of the item or scale beyond the .05 level of significance.

A structured procedure for the evaluation of the content validity of the instrument should be given to the experts. Experts selected must have specific criteria for deciding upon the relevance of the content to the concept. If the concept includes multiple dimensions, then criteria related to each dimension should also be supplied. According to the process defined by Lynn (1986), the content is quantified by use of the index of content validity. She notes that the authors of the index of content validity identify two limitations to the tool, but the method she proposes is presented as addressing these concerns. According to that procedure, a formula is applied to determine the number of experts needed and the proportion who must agree in order for content validity to be established. Each item, and the total scale, is quantified using the index of content validity. The experts identify areas that were omitted from the instrument, and items that do not achieve the required minimum agreement of the experts are eliminated or revised. Several items in the instrument may need to be evaluated more than once in order to establish sufficient content validity. In this case, the investigator, if using the same experts, waits for a period of 10 to 14 days between assessments. For further information on this process, see Lynn (1986). Content validity should not be an arbitrary decision; rather, it should include the application of rigorous criteria involving quantification.

Criterion-Related Validity

Criterion-related validity is at issue when an instrument is used to estimate some form of behavior that is external to the measuring instrument itself. The latter is often referred to as the criterion. There are two types of criterion-related validity: predictive validity and concurrent validity. *Predictive validity* refers to the extent to which an individual's future level of performance on the criterion can be predicted from his or her present performance on a specific measure. *Concurrent validity* refers to the extent to which a measure can be used to estimate an individual currently undergoing performance on the criterion.

The procedure for testing criterion-related validity is relatively straightforward. The researcher identifies the criterion variable and measures a sample of the population on both the predictor (the instrument) and criterion variables—a present criterion in concurrent validity and a future criterion in predictive validity. Scores of individuals' performance on the predictor and criterion variables are correlated, and this provides an index of the usefulness of the predictor variable in determining performance on the criterion for that specific population. The size of the correlation is a direct indicator of validity. Predictive validity is determined strictly by the degree of correlation between the two measures involved, and not by any other form of evidence. Nunnally (1978) notes that in most criterion-related situations, one can achieve only modest correlations between the criterion and the predictor tests because people are too complex to permit a more accurate estimate of their performance from any test materials. Nunnally cautions that one should interpret a validity coefficient in terms of the degree of possible improvement in performance that might be expected given an individual's score on a specific instrument.

Criterion-related validity is important mostly for making decisions about certain types of applied problems in the social sciences. It is very important in the case of evaluating people for a training program, assigning people to different types of classes, or making decisions concerning the management of people. The results from criterion-related validity testing are generalizable only to the target population studied. Also, the validity coefficients are relevant only to one point in time or to some specified later point; they are not generalizable beyond that specified time period.

A major problem with criterion-related validity is difficulty in obtaining a good criterion. The more abstract the concept, the less likely it is that one will be able to discover appropriate criteria for assessing or measuring it. Also, in some situations external criteria are simply not available. Often there are serious faults in the selection of a good criterion and there may well be limitations on the reliability and validity of the criterion measure. The criterion that should be used against a test score should be logically derived from the same concept the test is trying to tap and not an operationalization of some other concept (Knapp, 1985). The use of criterion-related validity has been criticized in the nursing research literature because the criterion selected as the external criterion for an abstract concept has been inappropriate. Nurse researchers have used other variables as an external criterion of the predictor variable that are theoretically related but are not a higher-level operationalization of the same concept as the predictor variable (Knapp, 1985). It has been noted that there has been some confusion between construct validity and criterion-related validity (Knapp, 1985). In construct validity all the variables used in the testing are on equal footing, whereas in criterion-related validity studies one of the variables has superior status (Knapp, 1985).

Construct Validity

Construct validity is concerned with the extent to which an instrument measures the concept or construct it was designed to measure (Kirshner & Guyatt, 1983). There are three major steps to testing construct validity. The first is the specification of the domain of observables related to the concept. The second is to support from research the extent to which the observables tend to measure the same concept, several different concepts, or many different concepts. The third is to subsequently perform studies of individual differences and/or controlled experiments to determine the extent to which the supposed measures of the concept produce results that are predictable from theory concerning the concept (Nunnally, 1978). The first two steps refer to the testing of validity by examining the internal association or pattern of interrelationships among the indicators designed to measure the concept. The third refers to validity testing by looking at the external association or the pattern of relationships between indicators designed to measure a concept and other variables.

Domain of observables. This refers to the attempt to support validity that occurs during scale development. As noted earlier in this chapter, concern with defining the concept and embedding it in theory is an important aspect of ensuring validity of the measure. Nunnally (1978) notes that this area is often poorly attended to; perusal of recent studies in nursing research (1981-1985) supports Nunnally's criticism.

Relations among observables. Nunnally (1978) notes that the way to test the adequacy of the identification of observables is to determine how well the measures of observables go together in empirical investigations. The quality of the work done in identifying the domain of observables will influence what occurs here. To determine the relationships among the variables, the researcher obtains scores for a sample of individuals on the measure, and then correlates different parts of the measure with other parts of the measure. An analysis of the correlations provides evidence on the extent to which all measures relate to the same concept.

Often the concept has been conceptualized as containing attributes, and these attributes were seen as separate dimensions of the concept. These attributes were defined and items were developed for each attribute or dimension. Factor analysis was then used to determine the relationship among the dimensions or the internal structure of the set of items. With the use of factor analysis, the researcher studies construct validity in terms of the internal consistency in which different aspects of a conceptual domain tend to correlate highly with one another and be similarly affected by experimental treatments.

Factor analysis as a construct validity technique is only as useful as the theory base upon which the concepts have been developed. If factor analysis is used when dimensions of the concept have not been conceptualized, as Nunnally (1978) puts it, "shotgun empiricism" is occurring. Factor analysis is useful when the theoretical structure of the concept has been well developed. Although factor analysis is used frequently in nursing research as a validity technique, often the conceptual basis upon which the factors have been proposed is poorly developed. Factor analysis functions as a construct validity technique only when the rotated factor structure produces factors consistent with those theoretically proposed in the conceptualization phase of instrument development.

If the factor analysis indicates that items cluster into multiple factors, which are interpretable according to the theoretically proposed dimensions, then it can be concluded that the measure reflects the number of different dimensions consistent with the concept. It does not, by these statistical manipulations, support validity via external association.

As Heise (1973) notes, there are no purely mathematical procedures for identifying conceptual variables with guaranteed theoretical validity. Internal association is not adequate to determine the construct validity of an instrument. That variables can group together and appear to be isomorphic with conceptual variables is not sufficient evidence for determining construct validity. Because the proposed number of factors emerge from the factor rotation does not assure isomorphism with the conceptual dimension. Zeller and Carmines (1980) note that there is an alternative interpretation of the factor solution. It may be that the dual dimensionality of the concept is a function of systematic measurement error and not a theoretically relevant dimension. A method artifact can systematically alter correlations among items and thus appear as a factor in a rotated factor solution. Therefore, factor analysis is not sufficient as a method of determining validity. In order to determine whether emerged factors are consistent with dimensions as theorized, the investigator must proceed from validity testing via internal association and proceed to testing validity via external association.

Relations between constructs. In this test of construct validity, sufficient evidence is that the supposed measures of the concept behave as expected (Nunnally, 1978). Support for the construct validity of an instrument occurs by determining the extent to which the measures fit in a lawful way into a network of relationships that are expected on the basis of theory. Testing for relationships among constructs is a method for determining construct validity via external association.

Construct validity is assessed within a given theoretical context. The external association that occurs is the relationship between the measure under development and the measure of another external concept to which it is supposedly theoretically related. It is impossible to validate the measure of a concept and its relationship to another concept unless a theoretical network exists to support these two measures. The logic of construct validity can be supported whether the concept is embedded in a systematized or a loose theory or framework or is linked with other concepts by even a few simple propositions. All that is required is several theoretically derived hypotheses involving the particulate concept under measurement. Zeller and Carmines (1980) note that construct validity is never confirmed, but is supported by predictions from multiple different studies. Construct validity requires a pattern of consistent findings involving multiple different studies across time performed by different researchers in regard to a variety of diverse theoretical variables.

Construct validity via external association is usually determined using three different methods: (1) discriminance approach, (2) causal inferences approach from experimental or nonexperimental data, and (3) the convergent/discriminant method.

Discriminance approach. Construct validity estimation by discriminance requires hypothesizing, from theoretical relational statements, differences expected among two groups of subjects hypothesized as extremely high and extremely low on the concept being measured by the instrument (Waltz et al., 1984). Determination of these groups and the rationale for why these groups should respond differently on the concept under measurement should be clearly supported by the theory surrounding the concept. The instrument is then administered to both groups and the differences in the scores are computed and examined. If the instrument performs as expected according to the theoretically proposed difference for these two groups, then support for the validity of this instrument may be proposed. But because the two groups may differ on multiple characteristics other than that being measured, one must remain sensitive to this possibility when claiming support for the validity of the instrument using the contrasting groups approach (Waltz et al., 1984). For an example of the use of this approach, see Mishel (1981, 1983) and Stevenson (1982). If significant differences are not found between the two groups even though there was a conceptual basis for the expectation of these differences, three possibilities exist: (1) The test is unreliable or perhaps not sufficiently sensitive; (2) the test, although reliable, is not a valid measure of the concept; or (3) there is a need for the researcher to reconceptualize the concept in terms of this population (Waltz et al., 1984). For an example of this third possibility, see Mishel (1983).

Causal inferences from experimental or nonexperimental data. Construct validity testing by an experimental or nonexperimental approach involves generating hypotheses from a theoretical or conceptual framework. The conceptual basis should be well developed, with a theoretical system that is as precise as possible. Operationalization of the other variables to be tested in the relational statements should be robust so as to reflect accurately the magnitude of the relationship. The researcher gathers data to test the hypotheses and then makes inferences on the basis of these findings as to whether or not the instrument under construction is adequate to explain the proposed relationships.

One of the ways to derive causal inferences is through use of experimental designs suitable for hypothesis testing. Nonexperimental methods for testing theoretical relationships among concepts include correlational descriptive studies and predictive modeling. Although predictive modeling uses a correlational descriptive design structure, not all correlational descriptive studies include predictive modeling. Predictive modeling involves theoretical model testing and requires a well-specified theoretical framework tested using multivariate data analysis methods (Hinshaw, 1984). On the other hand, correlational descriptive designs can be used to test relational statement from a looser theory or a few simple propositions. For an example of the use of predictive modeling for estimating construct validity, see Hinshaw, Gerber, Atwood, and Allen (1983).

Whichever method is used to test relational statements, a program of repeated testing should be planned to gauge the strength and generality of the relationships. One systematic procedure for investigating conceptual relationships is to begin testing in a tightly controlled setting, moving to progressively looser conditions to determine if the relationship persists. Specified relationships or a theoretical model of multiple relationships may behave differently under different conditions. Thus populations and contextual variables can be systematically varied to test the viability of the relationship under diverse conditions.

If the evidence relevant to conceptual relationships is negative, four different interpretations are possible. The first is that the instrument does not measure the intended concept. A second alternative is that the theoretical framework upon which the empirical prediction was based is incorrect. The third possibility is that the procedure used to test the empirical prediction was faulty. And finally, the negative evidence may be due to a lack of construct validity in some other variable in the analysis (Zeller & Carmines, 1980). Since there is no certain way to determine which of these explanations is correct, further programmatic testing is necessary. The determination of construct validity rests upon the gradual accumulation of evidence.

Convergent/discriminant method. The multitrait, multimethod matrix method involves the concepts of convergence and discriminance. *Convergence* refers to measuring the same concept using different methods and obtaining similar results. *Discriminance* refers to measuring different concepts using the same method and obtaining different results. Obtaining convergence and discriminance supports the construct validity of the instrument. This approach estimates trait versus method variance. If the correlations between different concepts measured by the same method are higher than correlations between the same concept measured by different methods, then a method artifact exists. Conversely, common trait variance exists if the correlation between measures of different concepts measured by the same method is lower than correlation between the same concept measured by different methods (Campbell & Fiske, 1959).

Because this approach requires measuring more than one concept as well as using more than one method to measure each concept, the several methods used to measure each concept must be appropriate to the conceptualization. Wherever possible, these methods should be completely independent of each other.

The correlations are cast into a matrix and examined to determine convergence and discriminance. The matrix consists of the reliability estimate for each measurement method used for each concept (reliability diagonal), correlations between two measures of each concept (validity diagonal), correlations between measures of two different concepts employing the same method (heterotrait-monomethod coefficients), and correlations between measures of different concepts measured by different methods (heterotrait-heteromethod coefficients). For further detail and an example of a matrix and its interpretation, see Campbell and Fiske (1959) or Waltz et al. (1984).

This approach has the advantage of using multiple operationalism in contrast to single operationalism. Multioperationalism provides a means for distinguishing common trait variance from method variance. Although an extremely valuable means of reliability and validity testing, the cost in time and money may reduce the appeal of the approach. Another consideration is that of the demands placed upon clinical populations who must complete multiple instruments at one point in time, which could potentially influence subjects' willingness to participate (Waltz et al., 1984).

CONCLUSION

The process of instrument development continuously involves controlling measurement error, thus enhancing the reliability and validity of the measure. In this chapter, the steps in instrument development have been linked to measurement error issues. The intent has been to highlight how measurement error can be reduced at each step in the instrument development process. A central idea in instrumentation is that it is more important to do everything possible to prevent measurement error from occurring rather than to try to assess the effects of measurement error after it has occurred.

REFERENCES

Aitken, R.C.B., & Zealley, A. K. (1970, August). Measurement of moods. *British Journal of Hospital Medicine,* pp. 215-224.

Anastasi, A. (1976). *Psychological testing* (4th ed.). New York: Macmillan.

Armstrong, G. D. (1981). Parametric statistics and ordinal data: A pervasive misconception. *Nursing Research, 30,* 60-62.

Baldree, K. S., Murphy, S. P., & Powers, M. J. (1982). Stress identification and coping patterns in patients on hemodialysis. *Nursing Research, 31*(2), 107-112.

Benoliel, J. Q., McCorkle, R., & Young, K. (1980). Development of a social dependency scale. *Research in Nursing and Health, 3,* 3-10.

Bohrnstedt, G. W. (1970). Reliability and validity assessment in attitude measurement. In G. F. Sinamers (Ed.), *Attitude measurement* (pp. 80-99). Chicago: Rand McNally.

Bond, A., & Lader, M. (1974). The use of analogue scales in rating subjective feelings. *British Journal of Medical Psychology, 47,* 211-218.

Burke, C. J. (1953). Additive scales and statistics. *Psychology Review, 60,* 73-75.

Campbell, D. T., & Fiske, D. W. (1959). Convergent and discriminant validation by the multitrait-multimethod matrix. *Psychological Bulletin, 56*(2), 81-104.

Carmines, E. G., & Zeller, R. A. (1979). *Reliability and validity assessment.* Beverly Hills, CA: Sage.

Cox, C. L. (1985). The health self-determinism index. *Nursing Research, 34*(3), 177-183.

Cranley, M. S. (1981). Development of a tool for the measurement of maternal attachment during pregnancy. *Nursing Research, 30*(5), 281-284.

Derogatis, L. R., & Spencer, P. M. (1984, May 15). Psychometric issues in the assessment of the cancer patient. *Cancer* (Suppl.), pp. 2228-2234.

Edwards, A. L., & Kilpatrick, F. P. (1948). A technique for construction of attitude scales. *Journal of Applied Psychology, 32,* 374-384.

Fox, R. N., & Ventura, M. R. (1983). Small-scale administration of instruments and procedures. *Nursing Research, 32*(2), 122-125.

Glaser, B. (1978). *Theoretical sensitivity.* Mill Valley, CA: Sociology Press.

Gordon, R. A. (1968). Issues in multiple regression. *American Journal of Sociology, 73,* 592-616.

Guilford, J. P. (1936). *Psychometric methods.* New York: McGraw Hill.

Heise, D. R. (1973-74). Some issues in sociological measurement. In H. Costner (Ed.), *Sociological methodology* (pp. 1-16). San Francisco: Jossey-Bass.

Hinshaw, A. S. (1984). Theoretical model testing: Full utilization of data. *Western Journal of Nursing Research, 6*(1), 5-10.

Hinshaw, A. S., & Atwood, J. R. (1982). A patient satisfaction instrument: Precision by replication. *Nursing Research, 31*(3), 170-175.

Hinshaw, A. S., Gerber, R. M., Atwood, J. R., & Allen, J. R. (1983). The use of predictive modeling to test nursing practice outcomes. *Nursing Research, 32*(1), 34-42.

Hoskins, C. N. (1981). Psychometrics in nursing research construction of an interpersonal conflict scale. *Research in Nursing and Health, 4,* 243-248.

Hoskins, C. N. (1983). Psychometrics in nursing research: Further development of the interpersonal conflict scale. *Research in Nursing and Health, 6*, 75-83.

Huskisson, E. C. (1974, November). Measurement of pain. *Lancet*, pp. 1127-1131.

Hymovich, D. P. (1983). The chronicity impact and coping instrument: Parent questionnaire. *Nursing Research, 32*(5), 275-281.

Isaac, S., & Michael, W. G. (1974). *Handbook in research and evaluation*. San Diego, CA: Knapp.

Jalowiec, A., & Powers, M. J. (1981). Stress and coping in hypertensive and emergency room patients. *Nursing Research, 30*(1), 10-16.

Kerlinger, F. N. (1986). *Foundations of behavioral research* (3rd ed.). New York: Holt, Rinehart & Winston.

Kirshner, B., & Guyatt, G. (1985). A methodological framework for assessing health indices. *Journal of Chronic Disease, 38*(1), 27-36.

Knapp, T. R. (1985). Validity, reliability, and neither. *Nursing Research, 34*(4), 251-256.

Labovitz, S. (1967). Some observations on measurement and statistics. *Social Forces, 46*(2), 151-160.

Lynn, M. R. (1986). The determination and quantification of content validity. *Nursing Research, 35*, 382-385.

Maxwell, C. (1978). Sensitivity and accuracy of the visual analogue scale: A psychophysical classroom experience. *British Journal of Clinical Pharmacology, 6*, 15-25.

McIver, J., & Carmines, E. (1978). *Unidimensional scaling*. Beverly Hills, CA: Sage.

Mishel, M. H. (1981). The measurement of uncertainty in illness. *Nursing Research, 30*(5), 258-263.

Mishel, M. H. (1983). Parents' perception of uncertainty concerning their hospitalized child. *Nursing Research, 32*(6), 324-330.

Murphy, S. P., Powers, M. J., & Jalowiec, A. (1985). Psychometric evaluation of the hemodialysis stressor scale. *Nursing Research, 34*(6), 368-371.

Nagel, E. (1974). Measurement Erkinnsnis II Bond, 1931. In G. Maranell (Ed.), *Scaling: A sourcebook for behavioral scientists*. Chicago: Aldine.

Norbeck, J. S., Lindsey, A. M., & Carrieri, V. L. (1981). The development of an instrument to measure social support. *Nursing Research, 30*(5), 264-269.

Nunnally, J. C. (1978). *Psychometric theory*. New York: McGraw-Hill.

Osgood, C. E., Suci, C. J., & Tannenbaum, P. H. (1957). *The measurement of meaning*. Urbana: University of Illinois Press.

Stevens, S. S. (1951). Mathematics, measurement and psychophysics. In S. S. Stevens (Ed.), *Handbook of experimental psychology*. New York: John Wiley.

Stevenson, J. S. (1982). Construction of a scale to measure load, power, and margin in life. *Nursing Research, 31*(4), 222-225.

Thurstone, L. L. (1927). The method of paired comparisons for social values. *Journal of Abnormal and Social Psychology, 21*, 384-400.

Thurstone, L. L. (1928). An experimental study of nationality preferences. *Journal of Genetic Psychology, 1*, 405-425.

Thurstone, L. L. (1929). Theory of attitude measurement. *Psychological Bulletin, 36*, 222-241.

Thurstone, L. L., & Chave, E. J. (1929). *The measurement of attitude*. Chicago: University of Chicago Press.

Title, C. R., & Hill, R. J. (1967). Attitude measurement and prediction of behavior: An evaluation of conditions and measurement techniques. *Sociometry, 30*, 199-213.

Torgerson, W. S. (1958). *Theory and methods of scaling*. New York: John Wiley.

Walker, L. O., & Avant, K. D. (1983). *Strategies for theory construction in nursing*. Norwalk, CT: Appleton-Century-Crofts.

Walker, L. O., & Avant, K. D. (1983). *Strategies for theory construction in nursing*. Norwalk, CT: Appleton-Century-Crofts.

Waltz, C. F., Strickland, O. L., & Lenz, E. R. (1984). *Measurement in nursing research*. Philadelphia: F. A. Davis.

Ware, J. E., Snyder, M. K., McClure, R. E., & Jarett, I. M. (1972). *The measurement of health concepts* (Tech. rep. No. HCP-72-5). Springfield, VA: U.S. Department of Commerce, National Technical Information Service.

Wolf, M. H., Putnam, S. M., James, S. A., & Stiles, W. B. (1978). The medical interview satisfaction scale: Development of a scale to measure patient perceptions of physician behavior. *Journal of Behavioral Medicine, 1*(4), 391-402.

Zeller, R. A., & Carmines, E. G. (1980). *Measurement in the social sciences*. London: Cambridge University Press.

13. The Pilot Study: One Key to Research Success

Nancy R. Lackey
Anita L. Wingate

Behind every successful piece of completed research stands a pilot study. In any basic research methodology course, students are told of the importance of a pilot study, but they are given little information on how to do one. Rarely is the actual conduct of a pilot study included in their assignments. It is questionable as to how much credence experienced nurse researchers give to pilot studies. A review of current nursing textbooks showed that approximately half of the authors refer to the term *pilot study*, but do not go into detail about how to conduct one. In those textbooks that list the term in the index, the actual coverage of the topic ranges from a brief entry in the glossary (Abdellah, Levine, & Levine, 1986) to a chapter delineating the definition and detailing the actual conduct of a study (Treece & Treece, 1986).

We recently completed collecting data for a qualitative study whose purpose was to determine the needs of noninstitutionalized cancer patients and their primary caregivers. The proposal included the statement that a pilot study would be completed before the actual study began. Little did we realize what a wealth of information we would obtain from our pilot study.

DEFINITION OF A PILOT STUDY

Our review of nursing research textbooks showed a number of terms that were used somewhat synonymously with the term *pilot study*:

pretest (Fox & Ventura, 1983; Treece & Treece, 1986), *small-scale study* (Fox & Ventura, 1983), and *exploratory study* (Dempsey & Dempsey, 1986; Woods & Catanzaro, 1988). According to Hogstel and Sayner (1986, p. 58), a pilot study is "a miniature version of the major research study and mimics or resembles the major research study in every detail." The terms *small-scale study*, *exploratory study*, and *preliminary study* are utilized identically to the term *pilot study* in most nursing research textbooks. When the term *preliminary study* is used, it most frequently refers to pilot study data incorporated into research grant proposals to "illustrate the investigators' competence to pursue the proposed project and relevant experience in studying the topic" (Woods & Catanzaro, 1988, p. 500).

The term *pretest*, when used in reference to pilot studies, has a slightly different connotation. Treece and Treece (1986) define a pilot study as a preliminary small-scale trial run of the research study that includes pretesting, which is the process of measuring the effectiveness of the instrument. The purpose of this pretesting of the instrument is to evaluate such factors as the length, wording, and validity of the instrument. Similarly, Fox and Ventura (1983) state two definitions of pretesting, one of which refers to the process of measuring the effectiveness of the instrument used to gather data, checking for reliability and preliminary indications of validity. Both of these sources also use the term *pretesting* as it is commonly used, meaning to gather baseline data about a sample for later comparisons in a posttest. For the purpose of this chapter, *pilot study* is defined as the exact miniature replica of a proposed major research study.

PHILOSOPHIES OF CONDUCTING PILOT STUDIES

From a general review of the literature, two basic philosophies about pilot studies become apparent. Sidman's (1960) philosophy suggests that an experiment is designated as a pilot study only after it has been performed and has proved to have technical flaws. He believes that any proposed major research study should be rigorously designed and conducted. If at any time during the conduct of the study a technical inadequacy is found, then the experiment becomes a pilot study and should not be published. If no flaws or procedural difficulties are encountered during the data collection or final written report, then the study is considered successful.

There are some advantages and disadvantages inherent in Sidman's (1960) philosophy. One advantage of this approach is that it allows the researcher to avoid spending time and money doing a pilot study that, because of its limited sample size, may not actually reveal lack of control over certain variables. Another advantage of this approach is that it allow the researcher to avoid depleting a limited population from which to draw a sample of subjects, for example, amyelotropic lateral sclerosis patients. The utilization of this philosophy is almost inevitable in conducting studies that examine phenomena associated with specified catastrophes such as the Coconut Grove fire or natural disasters, which, by their very nature, preclude the opportunity for pilot testing. A disadvantage of Sidman's philosophy is the expenditure of time, money, and effort in the execution of a major study that may prove to have serious flaws that might have been detected using a less costly pilot study. This becomes extremely problematic if grant funds have been used to conduct the large study.

A controversy related to this philosophy is whether or not a pilot study should be published. According to Sidman (1960), a study should be published only if no serious flaws have been recognized during the conduct of the study. He believes, however, that publication of a pilot study is justified if a technique is discovered that would be valuable to other researchers, of if new insights are developed about the research topic that have been alluded to in previous literature. Others agree that there are specific occasions when the total pilot study or selected parts of it should be published (Burns & Grove, 1987; Meyer & Heidgerken, 1962; Seaman & Verhonick, 1982).

The most commonly expressed philosophy about conducting a pilot study is that the whole major research proposal should be vigorously conducted on a small scale to search for defects in the methodology (Polit & Hungler, 1987; Treece & Treece, 1986). Other textbooks state that not only should methodology be pretested, but so should all of the components of the major study, such as instruments, directions, selection of subjects, and data recording forms (Hogstel & Sayner, 1986; Ort, 1981; Shelley, 1984). This philosophy is based on the assumption that the data collected during the pilot study will not be included in the analysis of the major study.

Advantages of this approach are that flaws in the large study may be detected without a large expenditure of time and money, and subsequent changes may improve the major proposal substantially. Nevertheless, it must be recognized that doing a pilot study with a limited sample may not, in fact, reveal all the flaws in the design, instruments, or methodology and will deplete the available population of potential subjects.

It has been our experience that a more plausible philosophy combines elements of both of the above. For example, if the researcher is experienced with the instruments and methodology used with a specific population, then certain parts of a pilot study may be unnecessary. Many sources emphasize pretesting the instrument or its administration, but may not advocate doing an entire pilot study (e.g., Fox & Ventura, 1983; Treece & Treece, 1986). Every researcher needs to evalutate diligently the major research study being proposed to determine which areas, if not all, need a "trial run." One pilot study may not be adequate; changes resulting from a completed pilot study may, in themselves, need to be "piloted" again. We believe that the main advantage of this philosophy is the eventual savings in time, effort, and expense. The main disadvantage in piloting is the possibility of overlooking major flaws that could seriously impair the outcome of a major study.

PURPOSE OF A PILOT STUDY

According to Ort (1981, p. 49), there are five basic purposes for conducting a pilot study:

(1) to determine the feasibility of the major study
(2) to identify problems in the research design
(3) to refine the data collection and analysis plan
(4) to test the instrument to be used in the major study
(5) to give the researcher some experience with the subjects, methodology, and instruments

CONDUCTING THE PILOT STUDY

Before the pilot study is undertaken, the entire major research proposal should be prepared and should have the approval of the institution's research review (human subjects) committee. Plans for the pilot study can either be included in the proposal that goes to the human subjects committee or written up separately and then submitted to the committee. Subjects in the pilot study must be guaranteed confidentiality and anonymity, just as they would in the major study.

Research Questions/Hypotheses

The research questions and/or hypotheses should be stated exactly as they will be for the proposed major study. The issue to be addressed here is whether or not the research questions/hypotheses will elicit the type of data the researcher desires. Actual data will be collected during the pilot study, and they should be analyzed carefully to ascertain whether or not they answer the research questions.

Subjects

Subjects selected for the pilot study should come from the same population from which the subjects in the proposed major study will be selected, although subjects included in the pilot study should not be included in the major study. The sample size will depend upon the overall size of the population, the amount of time the researcher has for the pilot study, and the cost. The sample must be large enough to detect flaws or weaknesses in the methodology. It is recommended that the pilot study sample be one-tenth of the size of the sample proposed for the major study (Treece & Treece, 1986). For example, if the sample size proposed for the major study is 60, then the sample size in the pilot study should be 6.

Instruments

A pilot study can be very useful in establishing the reliability and validity of an instrument. There are specific tests that can be built into the pilot study that measure the reliability and validity of an instrument. Also, the time it takes respondents to complete a questionnaire, survey, or research tool can be established in the pilot study. The researcher should ask the subjects to complete the instruments used in the study and to include comments about the instruments.

In our study, we used the Object Content Test, which is an unstructured, self-administered, paper-and-pencil test that can be administered to respondents either in a group or individually (Garretson, 1967). We structured our question after the examples accompanying the instrument. Initially, the wording was, "When I see the phrase 'needs of the cancer patient,' to me it means. . . ." During our pilot study, we learned that the way this was stated was confusing to the subjects. We changed it to read, "What are the needs of the noninstitutionalized cancer patient?" Our second pilot study demonstrated that the revised question elicited the types of responses that were appropriate for the research question. The instructions on the questionnaire asked the subjects to "go along fairly fast." During our pilot study, we were reminded that patients receiving radiation treatments or chemotherapy are fatigued and can do few things fast. We removed this statement from our directions, as the responses were more important than the time element.

Methodology

While conducting our pilot study, we became aware of a problem in the actual procedure. After selecting our subjects, we contacted them by phone, explained the study, and asked them if they would participate. If they consented, we then set up an appointment to deliver the questionnaire, demographic data sheets, and a self-addressed, stamped envelope in which they were to return the materials. During this visit to the home, the study was again explained and instructions were given about return of the completed materials.

During the pilot study, it became evident that the return rate was far below our expectations, even after telephone calls to the subjects to answer questions and to encourage them to complete and mail the materials. Three weeks into the pilot study, we realized that we were going to have inadequate responses with this procedure. Our revised procedure was to place an initial call to the subjects, as before, to describe the study and to ask them to participate. If they consented, we mailed the questionnaires, demographic data sheets, and instructions to them. We also informed them that we would call again in five days to make an appointment to come to their residence to collect their complete materials. We pilot tested these changes and learned that this procedure was more successful than the previous one. There was one flaw: the U.S. mail moved more slowly than we had anticipated. Therefore, we allowed a week rather than five days to establish the appointment for pickup of completed materials.

During the first pilot study, we realized that our record-keeping form was insufficient, as we were trying to match patients' data with those of their primary caregivers. Since this required a precise coding system, we revamped and enlarged our form and established a better coding system. These changes were then pilot tested to make sure that they would meet our needs with a large number of subjects.

Data Analysis

The researcher should be able to get an idea of what the data from the major study will look like at the end of the pilot study. Since the proposed statistical test should be included in the major proposed research study, the researcher should be able to tell if the proposed analysis is appropriate to either answer the research question or accept or reject the hypothesis. The researcher should be able to speculate from the data collected in the pilot study whether or not the statistical test will do this. The kind of data generated in the pilot study may suggest the need for additional or different kinds of data analysis.

EVALUATING THE RESULTS OF THE PILOT STUDY

The researcher must remember that not all of the flaws of a major proposed research study will show up in a pilot study, because a pilot study uses a small sample size, is an artificial situation, and has a limited scope (Hogstel & Sayner, 1986; Treece & Treece, 1986). In evaluating the results of the pilot study, the researcher must identify the weaknesses and strengths of the research questions/hypotheses, methodology, and analysis. The results elicited in the pilot study should be given careful consideration.

Some of the major questions the researcher should ask at this time are as follows: What weaknesses have appeared in the proposed major research study prior to its implementation? Based on the results of the pilot study, is the proposed major research study warranted? Will the results of the proposed major research study justify the proposed cost and time involved? If the evaluation of the results of the pilot study determines that a number of changes or a major methodological change needs to be made in the larger study, then it is advisable to conduct a second pilot study that incorporates these changes.

SUMMARY

Many researchers do not conduct pilot studies, mainly because of the time involvement they require. However, more grant applications are now requiring evidence of a pilot study. No matter how diligent a researcher is in planning a proposed major research study, there will always be unanticipated flaws. If these flaws are corrected before the initiation of the major research study, the researcher's time, money, and efforts are more likely to be rewarded with meaningful findings in the larger project.

REFERENCES

Abdellah, F. G., Levine, E., & Levine, B. S. (1986) *Better patient care through nursing research*. New York: Macmillan.

Burns, N., & Grove, S. K. (1987). *The practice of nursing research: Conduct, critique and utilization*. Philadelphia: W. B. Saunders.

Dempsey, P. A., & Dempsey, A. D. (1986). *The research process in nursing*. Boston: Jones & Bartlett.

Fox, R. N., & Ventura, M. R. (1983). Small-scale administration of instruments and procedures. *Nursing Research, 32*(2), 122-125.

Garretson, W. S. (1967). The consensual definition of social objects. In J. G. Morris & B. N. Meltzer (Eds.). *Symbolic interaction* (pp. 337-342). Boston: Allyn & Bacon.

Hogstel, M. O., & Sayner, N. C. (1986). *Nursing research*. New York: McGraw-Hill.

Meyer, B., & Heidgerken, L. E. (1962). *Introduction to research in nursing*. Philadelphia: J. B. Lippincott.

Ort, S. V. (1981). Research design: Pilot study. In S. D. Krampitz & N. Pavlovich (Eds.), *Reading for nursing research*. St. Louis: C. V. Mosby.

Polit, D. F., & Hungler, B. P. (1987). *Nursing research*. Philadelphia: J. B. Lippincott.

Seaman, C., & Verhonick, P. (1982). *Research methods*. Norwalk, CT: Appleton-Century-Crofts.

Shelley, S. I. (1984) *Research methods in nursing and health*. Boston: Little, Brown.

Sidman, M. (1960). Pilot studies. In M. Sidman, *Tactics of scientific research* (pp. 217-223). New York: Basic Books.

Treece, E. W., & Treece, J. W. (1986). *Elements of research in nursing*. St. Louis: C. V. Mosby.

Woods, N. F., & Catanzaro, M. (1988). *Nursing research: Theory and practice*. St. Louis: C. V. Mosby.

Recommended Readings

Experimental Designs

Clinton, J. (1985). Couvade: Patterns, predictors, and nursing management—A research proposal submitted to the Division of Nursing. *Western Journal of Nursing Research, 7*(2), 121-143.

Gordon, V. C., & Ledray, L. E. (1986). Growth-support intervention for the treatment of women of middle years. *Western Journal of Nursing Research, 8*(3), 263-283.

King, K. B., Norsen, L. H., Robertson, R. K., & Hicks, G. L. (1987). Patient management of pain medication after cardiac surgery. *Nursing Research, 36*(3), 145-150.

Riegel, B. J., & Dracup, K. (1986). Teaching nurses priority setting for patients with pain of acute myocardial infarction. *Western Journal of Nursing Research, 8*(3), 306-320.

Shelley, S. I., Zahorchak, R. M., & Gambrill, C. D. S. (1987). Aggressiveness of nursing care for older patients and those with do-not-resuscitate orders. *Nursing Research, 36*(3), 157-162.

Quasi-Experimental Designs

Boyer, D. B., & Vidyasagar, D. (1987). Serum indirect bilirubin levels and meconium passage in early fed normal newborns. *Nursing Research, 36*(3), 174-178.

Keefe, M. (1987). Comparison of neonatal nighttime sleep-wake patterns in nursery versus rooming-in environments. *Nursing Research, 36*(3), 140-144.

Kirchhoff, K. T., Rebenson-Piano, M., & Patel, M. K. (1984). *Mean arterial pressure readings: Variations with positions and transducer level.* Unpublished manuscript.

Owen, B. D. (1985). The lifting process and back injury in hospital nursing personnel. *Western Journal of Nursing Research, 7*(4), 445-459.

Comparative Designs

Glascock, J., Webster-Stratton, C., & McCarthy, A. M. (1985). Infant and preschool well-child care: Master's- and nonmaster's-prepared pediatric nurse practitioners. *Nursing Research, 34*(1), 39-43.

LaMontagne, L. L. (1987). Children's preoperative coping: Replication and extension. *Nursing Research, 36*(3), 163-167.

McLaughlin, F., Cesa, T., Johnson, H., Lemons, M., Anderson, S., Larson, P., Gibson, J., & Delucchi, K. (1979). Nurse practitioners', public health nurses' and physicians' performance on clinical simulation tests. *Western Journal of Nursing Research, 1*(4), 273-295.

Mynatt, S. (1985). Empathy in faculty and students in different types of nursing preparation programs. *Western Journal of Nursing Research, 7*(3), 333-348.

Ouellette, M. D., MacVicar, M. G., Harlan, J. (1986). Relationship between percent body fat and menstrual patterns in athletes and non-athletes. *Nursing Research, 35*(6), 330-333.

Reed, P. G. (1986). Developmental resources and depression in the elderly. *Nursing Research, 35*(6), 368-378.

Taylor, M. S., & Covaleski, M. A. (1985). Predicting nurses' turnover and internal transfer behavior. *Nursing Research, 34*(4), 237-241.

Correlational Designs

Brown, N., Muhlenkamp, A., Fox, L., & Osborn, M. (1983). The relationship among health beliefs, health values, and health promotion activity. *Western Journal of Nursing Research, 5*(2), 155-164.

Damrosch, S. (1982). More than skin deep: Relationship between perceived physical attractiveness and nursing students' assignments. *Western Journal of Nursing Research, 4*(4), 423-434.

Fink, A., & Koseocoff, J. (1985). *How to conduct surveys: A step-by-step guide.* Beverly Hills, CA: Sage.

Hilbert, G. A. (1985). Spouse support and myocardial infarction patient compliance. *Nursing Research, 34*(4), 217-220.

Janson-Bjerklie, S., Ruma, S. S., Stulbarg, M., & Carrieri, V. K. (1987). Predictors of dyspnea intensity in asthma. *Nursing Research, 36*(3), 179-183.

Ketefian, S. (1985). Professional and bureaucratic role conceptions and moral behavior among nurses. *Nursing Research, 34*(4), 248-253.

Laffrey, S. C. (1985). Health behavior choice as related to self-actualization and health conception. *Western Journal of Nursing Research, 7*(3), 279-300.

Muhlenkamp, A. F., & Sayles, J. A. (1986). Self-esteem, social support, and positive health practices. *Nursing Research, 35*(6), 334-338.

Norbeck, J. S. (1985). Types and sources of social support for managing job stress in critical care nursing. *Nursing Research, 34*(4), 225-230.

Rudy, E. B., & Estok, P. J. (1983). Intensity of jogging: Its relationship to selected physical and psychosocial variables in women. *Western Journal of Nursing Research, 5*(4), 325-336.

Wernet, P. Z., & Weiss, S. J. (1987). Health locus of control and preventive health behavior. *Western Journal of Nursing Research, 9*(2), 160-174.

Descriptive Designs

Aamodt, A. (1982). Examining ethnography for nursing researchers. *Western Journal of Nursing Research, 4*(2), 209-222.

Agar, M. H. (1980). *The professional stranger: An informal introduction to ethnography.* New York: Academic Press.

Agar, M. H. (1986). *Speaking of ethnography.* Beverly Hills, CA: Sage.

Bullough, B., Bullough, V., & Smith, R. W. (1985). Masculinity and femininity in transvestite, transsexual and gay males. *Western Journal of Nursing Research, 7*(3), 317-332.

Carrieri, V. K., & Janson-Bjerklie, S. (1986). Strategies patients use to manage the sensation of dyspnea. *Western Journal of Nursing Research, 8*(3), 284-305.

Cohen, F. S. (1982). Childbirth belief and practice in a Garifuna (Black Carib) village on the north coast of Honduras. *Western Journal of Nursing Research, 4*(2), 193-208.

Crane, J. G., & Angrosino, M. V. (1985). *Field projects in anthropology: A student handbook*. Prospect Heights, IL: Waveland.

Cressler, D. L., & Tomlinson, P. S. (1988). Nursing research and the discipline of ethological science. *Western Journal of Nursing Research, 10*(6), 743-756.

Ellen, R. F. (1984). *Ethnographic research: A guide to general conduct*. London: Academic Press.

Evaneshko, V., & Kay, M. A. (1982). The ethnoscience research technique. *Western Journal of Nursing Research, 4*(1), 49-64.

Foxall, M. J., Ekberg, J. Y., & Griffith, N. (1985). Adjustment patterns of chronically ill middle-aged persons and spouses. *Western Journal of Nursing Research, 7*(4), 425-444.

Germain, C. (1986). Ethnography: The method. In P. L. Munhall and C. J. Oiler (Eds.), *Nursing research: A qualitative perspective* (pp. 147-162). Norwalk, CT: Appleton-Century-Crofts.

Hammersley, M., & Atkinson, P. (1983). *Ethnography: Principles in practice*. New York: Tavistock.

Karraker, K. H. (1986). Adult attention to infants in a newborn nursery. *Nursing Research, 35*(6), 358-363.

Kayser-Jones, J. (1979). Care of the institutionalized aged in Scotland and the United States. *Western Journal of Nursing Research, 1*(3), 190-200.

Kerr, J. A. C. (1986). Interpersonal distance of hospital staff. *Western Journal of Nursing Research, 8*(3), 350-364.

Lofland, J. (1971). *Analyzing social settings*. Belmont, CA: Wadsworth.

McCall, G. J., & Simmons, J. L. (Eds.). (1969). *Issues in participant observation: A text and reader*. Reading, MA: Addison-Wesley.

Meisenhelder, J. B., & Meservey, P. M. (1987). Childbearing over thirty: Description and satisfaction with mothering. *Western Journal of Nursing Research, 9*(4), 527-541.

Miles, M. B., & Huberman, A. M. (1984). *Qualitative data analysis: A sourcebook of new methods*. Beverly Hills, CA: Sage.

Reimer, T. T. (1982). Barriers to health care: Variations in interpretation of Appalachian client behavior by Appalachian and non-Appalachian health professionals. *Western Journal of Nursing Research, 4*(2), 179-192.

Roberson, M. (1987). Folk health beliefs of health professionals. *Western Journal of Nursing Research, 9*(2), 257-263.

Shamansky, S. L., Schilling, L. S., & Holbrook, T. L. (1985). Determining the market for nurse practitioner services: The New Haven experience. *Nursing Research, 34*(4), 242-247.

Spradley, J. P. (1979). *The ethnographic interview*. New York: Holt, Rinehart & Winston.

Spradley, J. P. (1980). *Participant observation*. New York: Holt, Rinehart & Winston.

Spradley, J. P., & McCurdy, D. W. (1972). The cultural experience: Ethnography in complex society. Chicago: Science Research Associates.

Tripp-Reimer, T. (1986). Health Heritage Project: A research proposal submitted to the Division of Nursing. *Western Journal of Nursing Research, 8*(2), 207-224.

Whiting, J. W. M., et al. (1966). *Field guide for a study of socialization*. New York: John Wiley.

Wilson, H. (1985). *Research in nursing*. Menlo Park, CA: Addison-Wesley.

Additional Readings in Descriptive Research

Aamodt, A. M. (1982). Examining ethnography for nurse researchers. *Western Journal of Nursing Research, 4*(2), 209-221.

Aamodt, A. M. (1983). Problems in doing nursing research: Developing criteria for evaluating qualitative research. *Western Journal of Nursing Research, 5*(4), 398-402.

Abraham, I., & Schultz, S., II. (1983). Univariate statistical models for meta-analysis. *Nursing Research, 32*(5), 312-315.

Allison, P. D. (1984). *Life event history analysis: Regression for longitudinal event data.* Beverly Hills, CA: Sage.

American Nurses Association. (1985). *Human rights guidelines for nurses in clinical and other research* (Document No. D-46 5M). Kansas City, MO: Author.

Andreoli, K. G., & Thompson, C. E. (1977). The nature of science in nursing. *Image, 9*(2), 32-37.

Armiger, B., Sr. (1977). Ethics of nursing research: Profile, principles, perspective. *Nursing Research, 26*(5), 330-336.

Babbie, E. (1973). *Survey research methods.* Belmont, CA: Wadsworth.

Baer, E. D. (1979). Philosophy provides the rationale for nursing's multiple research directions. *Image, 11*(3), 72-74.

Baer, E. D. (1985). Nursing's divided house: An historical view. *Nursing Research, 34*(1), 32-38.

Batey, M. V. (1977). Conceptualization: Knowledge and logic guiding empirical research. *Nursing Research,24*(5), 324-329.

Beck, C. T. (1984). Subject mortality: Is it inevitable? *Western Journal of Nursing Research, 6*(3), 331-339.

Becker, C. H. (1983). A conceptualization of concept. *Nursing Papers, 15*(2), 51-58.

Benner, P. (1984). *From novice to expert: Excellence and power in clinical practice.* Menlo Park, CA: Addison-Wesley.

Benoliel, J. Q. (1984). Advancing nursing science: Quantitative approaches. *Western Journal of Nursing Research, 6*(3), 1-8.

Blalock, H. M. (1982). *Conceptualization and measurement in the social sciences.* Beverly Hills, CA: Sage.

Brogan, D. R. (1981). Choosing an appropriate statistical test for a nursing research hypothesis or question. *Western Journal of Nursing Research, 3*(4), 337-368.

Bullough, B., Bullough, V., & Smith, R. W. (1985). Masculinity and femininity in transvestite, transsexual and gay males. *Western Journal of Nursing Research, 7*(3), 317-332.

Burns, N., & Grove, S. K. (1987). *The practice of nursing research, conduct, critique and utilization.* Philadelphia: W. B. Saunders.

Campbell, D. T., & Stanley, J. C. (1966). *Experimental and quasi-experimental designs for research.* Chicago: Rand McNally.

Carrieri, V. K., & Janson-Bjerklie, S. (1986). Strategies patients use to manage the sensation of dypnea. *Western Journal of Nursing Research, 8*(3), 284-305.

Chinn, P. L. (1986). *Nursing research methodology: Issues and implementation.* Rockville, MD: Aspen.

Christy, T. E. (1975). The methodology of historical research: A brief introduction. *Nursing Research, 24*(3), 189-192.

Clinton, J., Beck, R., Radjenovic, D., Taylor, L., Westlake, S., & Wilson, S. E. (1986). Time series design in clinical research: Human issues. *Nursing Research, 35*(3), 188-191.

Cohen, F. S. (1982). Childbirth belief and practice in Garifuna (Black Carib) village on the north coast of Honduras. *Western Journal of Nursing Research, 4*(2), 193-208.

Cohen, M. X., & Loomis, M. E. (1985). Linguistic analysis of questionnaire responses: Methods of coping with work stress. *Western Journal of Nursing Research, 7*(3), 357-366.

Cook, T. D., & Campbell, D. T. (Eds.). (1979). *Quasi-experimentation: Design and analysis issues for field settings.* Chicago: Rand McNally.

Cronbach, L. J., & Meehl, P. E. (1955). Construct validity in psychological tests. *Psychological Bulletin, 52*(4), 281-302.

Davis, A. (1985). Informed consent: How much information is enough? *Nursing Outlook, 33*(1), 40-42.

Diers, D. (1979). *Research in nursing practice.* Philadelphia: J. B. Lippincott.

Dobbert, M. L. (1982). *Ethnographic research: Theory and application for modern schools and societies.* New York: Praeger.

Downs, F. S., & Fleming, J. W. (1979). *Issues in nursing research.* New York: Appleton-Century-Crofts.

Egger, M. J., & Miller, J. R. (1984). Testing for experimental effects in the pretest-posttest design. *Nursing Research, 33*(5), 306-312.

Evaneshko, V., & Kay, M. A. (1982). The ethnoscience research techniques. *Western Journal of Nursing Research, 4*(1), 49-63.

Ferketich, L. S., & Verron, J. A. (1984). Residual analysis for causal model assumptions. *Western Journal of Nursing Research, 6*(1), 41-76.

Fisher, R. A. (1935). *The designs of experiments.* New York: Hafner.

Fitzpatrick, M. L. (1978). *Historical studies in nursing.* New York: Teachers College Press.

Fleming, J. W., & Hayter, J. (1974). Reading research reports critically. *Nursing Outlook, 22*(3), 172-175.

Glaser, B. G. (1978). *Theoretical sensitivity.* Mill Valley, CA: Sociology Press.

Glaser, B. G., & Strauss, A. L. (1967). *The discovery of grounded theory: Strategies for qualitative research.* Chicago: Sociology Press.

Goetz, J. P., & LeCompte, M. D. (1984). *Ethnography and qualitative design in educational research.* Orlando, FL: Academic Press.

Goodwin, L. D. (1984). The use of power estimation in nursing research. *Nursing Research, 33*(2), 118-120.

Gortner, S. R. (1975). Research for practice profession. *Nursing Research, 24*(3), 193-197.

Hinshaw, A. S. (1984). Theoretical model testing: Full utilization of data. *Western Journal of Nursing Research, 6*(1), 5-10.

Ihde, D. (1977). *Experimental phenomenology: An introduction.* New York: G. P. Putnam.

James, L. R., Mulaik, S. A., & Brett, J. M. (1982). *Causal analysis: Assumptions, models, and data.* Beverly Hills, CA: Sage.

Kayser-Jones, J. (1979). Care of the institutionalized aged in Scotland and the United States. *Western Journal of Nursing Research, 1*(3), 190-200.

Kerlinger, F. N. (1973). *Foundations of behavioral research.* New York: Holt, Rinehart & Winston.

Kerr, J. A. C. (1986). Interpersonal distance of hospital staff. *Western Journal of Nursing Research, 8*(3), 350-364.

Kim, J.-O., & Mueller, C. W. (1978a). *Introduction to factor analysis: What it is and how to do it.* Beverly Hills, CA: Sage.

Kim, J.-O., & Mueller, C. W. (1978b). *Factor analysis: Statistical methods and practical issues.* Beverly Hills, CA: Sage.

Krampitz, S. D., & Pavlovich, N. (Eds.). (1981). *Readings for nursing research.* St. Louis: C. V. Mosby.

Levy, P. S., & Lemsbow, S. (1980). *Sampling for health professionals.* Belmont, CA: Lifetime Learning.

Lofland, J. (1971). *Analyzing social settings.* Belmont, CA: Wadsworth.

Ludemann, R. (1979). The paradoxical nature of nursing research. *Image, 11*(1), 2-8.

Lynn, M. R. (1985). Reliability estimates: Use and disuse. *Nursing Research, 34*(4), 254-256.

McCleary, R., & Hay, R. A. (1980). *Applied time-series analysis for the social sciences.* Beverly Hills, CA: Sage.

McDowell, D., McCleary, R., Meidinger, E. E., & Hay, R. A. (1980). *Interrupted time series analysis.* Beverly Hills, CA: Sage.

McIver, J. P., & Carmines, E. G. (1981). *Unidimensional scaling.* Beverly Hills, CA: Sage.

Metzger, B. L., & Schultz, S. (1982). Time series analysis: An alternative for nursing. *Nursing Research, 31*(6), 375-378.

Meisenhelder, J. B., & Meservey, P. M. (1987). Childbearing over thirty: Description and satisfaction with mothering. *Western Journal of Nursing Research, 9*(4), 527-541.

Miller, T. W. (1981). Life events scaling: Clinical methodological issues. *Nursing Research, 30*(5), 316-320.

Munhall, P., & Oiler, C. J. (Eds.). (1986). *Nursing research: A qualitative perspective.* Norwalk, CT: Appleton-Century-Crofts.

Myers, S. T. (1982). The search for assumptions. *Western Journal of Nursing Research, 4*(1), 91-98.

Newton, M. E. (1965). The case for historical research. *Nursing Research, 14*(1), 20-26.

Nieswiadomy, R. M. (1987). *Foundations of nursing research.* Norwalk, CT: Appleton-Century-Crofts.

O'Flynn, A. I. (1982). Meta-analysis. *Nursing Reseach, 31*(5), 314-316.

Oiler, C. (1982). The phenomenological approach in nursing research. *Nursing Research, 31*(3), 178-181.

Omery, A. (1983). Phenomenology: A method for nursing research. *Advances in Nursing Science, 5*(2), 49-63.

Parse, R. R., Coyne, A. B., & Smith, M. J. (1985). *Nursing research: Qualitative methods.* Bowie, MD: Brady.

Patton, M. (1980). *Qualitative evaluation methods.* Beverly Hills, CA: Sage.

Reimer, T. T. (1982). Barriers to health care: Variations in interpretation of Appalachian client behavior by Appalachian and non-Appalachian health professionals. *Western Journal of Nursing Research, 4*(2), 179-192.

Roberson, M. (1987). Folk health beliefs of health professionals. *Western Journal of Nursing Research, 9*(2), 257-263.

Selltiz, C., Wrightsman, L. S., & Cook, S. W. (1981). *Research methods in social relations* (4th ed.). New York: Holt, Rinehart & Winston.

Shamansky, S. L., Schilling, L. S., & Holbrook, T. L. (1985). Determining the market for nurse practitioner services: The New Haven experience. *Nursing Research, 34*(4), 242-247.

Shelley, S. I. (1984). *Research methods in nursing and health.* Boston: Little, Brown.

Siegel, S. (1956). *Nonparametric statistics for the behavioral sciences.* New York: McGraw-Hill.

Simms, L. M. (1981). The grounded theory approach in nursing research. *Nursing Research, 30*(6), 356-359.

Smith, J. K. (1983). Quantitative versus qualitative research: An attempt to clarify the issue. *Educational Researcher, 12*(3), 6-13.

Spector, P. E. (1981). *Research designs.* Beverly Hills, CA: Sage.

Stern, P. N. (1980). Grounded theory methodology: Its uses and processes. *Image, 12*(1), 20-23.

Suchman, E. A. (1967). *Evaluative research principles and practice in public service and social action programs.* New York: Russell Sage Foundation.

Swanson, J. M., & Chenitz, W. C. (1982). Why qualitative research in nursing? *Nursing Outlook, 30*(4), 241-245.

Tilden, V. P., & Tilden, S. (1985). The participant philosophy in nursing science. *Image*, 17(3), 881-890.

Tripp-Reimer, T. (1986). Health Heritage Project: A research proposal submitted to the Division of Nursing. *Western Journal of Nursing Research*, 8(2), 207.

Volicer, B. J. (1984). *Multivariate statistics for nursing research*. New York: Grune & Stratton.

Waltz, C. F., & Bausell, R. B. (1981). *Nursing research: Design, statistics and computer analysis*. Philadelphia: F. A. Davis.

Waltz, C. F., Strickland, O. L., & Lenz, E. R. (1984). *Measurement in nursing research*. Philadelphia: F. A. Davis.

Ward, M. J., & Lindeman, C. (1979). *Instruments for measuring nursing practice and other health care variables* (DHEW Publication Nos. HRA 78-53, HRA 78-54). Washington, DC: Government Printing Office.

Watson, A. B. (1982). Informed consent of special subjects. *Nursing Research*, 31(1), 43-47.

Werley, H. H., Fitzpatrick, J. J., & Taunton, R. L. (Eds.). (1983-1986). *Annual review of nursing research* (4 vols.). New York: Springer.

Whiting, J. W. M., et al. (1966). *Field guide for a study of socialization*. New York: John Wiley.

Wilson, H. S. (1985). *Research in nursing*. Menlo Park, CA: Addison-Wesley.

Wooldridge, P. J., Leonard, R. C., & Skipper, J. K. (1978). *Methods of clinical experimentation to improve patient care*. St. Louis: C. V. Mosby.

Exploratory Designs

Aamodt, A. (1981). Neighboring: Discovering support systems among Norwegian-American women. In D. A. Messerschmidt (Ed.), *Anthropologists at home: Methods and issues in the study of one's own society* (pp. 133-152). New York: Cambridge University Press.

Agar, M. H. (1980). *The professional stranger: An informal introduction to ethnography*. New York: Academic Press.

Agar, M. H. (1986). *Speaking of ethnography*. Beverly Hills, CA: Sage.

Anderson, J. (1989). The phenomenological perspective. In J. Morse (Ed.), *Qualitative nursing research: A contemporary dialogue* (pp. 15-26). Rockville, MD: Aspen.

Anderson, N. L. (1987). *Doing time and making choices: The anthropology of pregnancy resolution decisions in juvenile detention*. Unpublished doctoral dissertation, University of California, Los Angeles.

Artinian, B. (1982). Conceptual mapping: Development of the strategy. *Western Journal of Nursing Research*, 4(4), 379-394.

Bogdan, R., & Taylor, S. J. (1974). *Introduction to qualitative research methods: A phenomenological approach to the social sciences*. New York: John Wiley.

Brinberg, D., & McGrath, J. E. (1985). *Validity and the research process*. Beverly Hills, CA: Sage.

Bruyn, S. T. (n.d.). *The human perspective in sociology: The methodology of participant observation*. Englewood Cliffs, NJ: Prentice-Hall.

Cobb, A. K., & Hagemaster, J.N. (1987). Ten criteria for evaluating qualitative research proposals. *Journal of Nursing Education*, 26(4), 138-143.

Crane, J. G., & Angrosino, M. V. (1984). *Field projects in anthropology: A student handbook* (2nd ed.). Prospect Heights, IL: Waveland.

Dean, J. P., & Whyte, W. F. (1969). How do you know if the infomant is telling the truth? In G. J. McCall & J. L. Simmons (Eds.), *Issues in participant observation: A text and reader* (pp. 105-115). Reading, MA: Addison-Wesley.

Dobbert, M. L. (1982). *Ethnographic research: Theory and application for modern schools and societies*. New York: Praeger.

Ellen, R. F. (1984). *Ethnographic research: A guide to general conduct.* New York: Academic Press.

Field, P. A., & Morse, J. M. (1985). *Nursing research: The application of qualitative approaches.* Rockville, MD: Aspen.

Fielding, N. G., & Fielding, J. L. (1986). *Linking data.* Beverly Hills, CA: Sage.

Fink, A., & Koseocoff, J. (1985). *How to conduct surveys: A step-by-step guide.* Beverly Hills, CA: Sage.

Gardner, K. G., & Wheeler, E. C. (1987). Patients' perceptions of support. *Western Journal of Nursing Research, 9*(1), 115-131.

Garfinkel, H. (1967). *Studies in ethnomethodology.* Englewood Cliffs, NJ: Prentice-Hall.

Germain, C. (1986). Ethnography: The method. In P. L. Munhall & C. J. Oiler (Eds.), *Nursing Research: A qualitative perspective* (pp. 147-162). Norwalk, CT: Appleton-Century-Crofts.

Goetz, J. P., & LeCompte, M. D. (1984). *Ethnography and qualitative design in educational research.* Orlando, FL: Academic Press.

Hammersley, M., & Atkinson, P. (1983). *Ethnography: Principles in practice.* New York: Tavistock.

Hunter, D. E., & Foley, M. B. (1976). *Doing anthropology: A student centered approach to cultural anthropology.* New York: Harper & Row.

Jackson, B. (1987). *Fieldwork.* Chicago: University of Illinois Press.

Johnson, J. M. (1975). *Doing field research.* New York: Free Press.

Johnson-Saylor, M. T. (1986). An exploratory study of the experience of resentment. *Western Journal of Nursing Research, 8*(1), 49-62.

Kirk, J., & Miller, M. L. (1986). *Reliability and validity in qualitative research.* Beverly Hills, CA: Sage.

Knafl, K. A. (1985). How families manage a pediatric hospitalization. *Western Journal of Nursing Research, 7*(2), 151-176.

Knafl, K. A. (Ed.) (1988). Qualitative research [Special issue]. *Western Journal of Nursing Research, 10*(2).

Krippendorf, K. (1980). *Content analysis: An introduction to its methodology.* Beverly Hills, CA: Sage.

Kus, R. J. (1985). Stages of coming out: An ethnographic approach. *Western Journal of Nursing Research, 7*(2), 177-198.

Leiter, K. (1980). *A primer on ethnomethodology.* New York: Oxford University Press.

Lincoln, Y. S., & Guba, E. G. (1985). *Naturalistic inquiry.* Beverly Hills, CA: Sage.

McCall, G. J., & Simmons, J. L. (Eds.). (1969). *Issues in participant observation: A text and reader.* Reading, MA: Addison-Wesley.

Mehan, H., & Wood, H. *The reality of ethnomethodology.* New York: John Wiley.

Miles, M. B., & Huberman, A. M. (1984). *Qualitative data analysis: A sourcebook of new methods.* Beverly Hills, CA: Sage.

Morgan, G. (Ed.). *Beyond method: Strategies for social research.* Beverly Hills, CA: Sage.

Munhall, P. L., & Oiler, C. J. (Eds.). (1986). *Nursing research: A qualitative perspective.* Norwalk, CT: Appleton-Century-Crofts.

Norris, C. M. (1975). Restlessness: A nursing phenomenon in search of meaning. *Nursing Outlook, 23*(2), 103-107.

Pelto, P. J., & Pelto, G. H. (1978). *Anthropological research: The structure of inquiry* (2nd ed.). Cambridge: Cambridge University Press.

Punch, M. (1986). *The politics and ethics of fieldwork.* Beverly Hills, CA: Sage.

Saylor, M. T. J. (1986). An exploratory study of the experience of resentment. *Western Journal of Nursing Research, 8*(1), 49-62.

Schwartz, H., & Jacobs, J. (1979). *Qualitative sociology: A method in the madness.* New York: Free Press.

Spradley, J. P. (1979). *The ethnographic interview.* New York: Holt, Rinehart & Winston.

Spradley, J. P., & McCurdy, D. W. (1972). *The cultural experience: Ethnography in complex society.* Chicago: Science Research Associates.

Stewart, D. W. (1984). *Secondary research: Information sources and methods.* Beverly Hills, CA: Sage.

Swanson-Kauffman, K. M. (1986, April). A combined qualitative methodology for nursing research. *Advances in Nursing Science,* pp. 58-69.

Van Maanen, J., Dabbs, J. M., Jr., & Faulkner, R. R. (1984). *Varieties of qualitative research.* Beverly Hills, CA: Sage.

Van Manen, M. (1984). *"Doing" phenomenological research and writing: An introduction* (Monograph No. 7). Alberta: University of Alberta, Faculty of Education, Department of Secondary Education.

Wax, T H. (1971). *Doing fieldwork: Warnings and advice.* Chicago: University of Chicago Press.

Werner, O., & Schoepfle, G.M. (1987). *Systematic fieldwork* (2 vols.). Newbury Park, CA: Sage.

Whyte, W. F. (1955). *Street corner society: The social structure of an Italian slum.* Chicago: University of Chicago Press.

Whyte, W. F. (1984). *Learning from the field: A guide from experience.* Beverly Hills, CA: Sage.

Yin, R. K. (1984). *Case study research: Design and methods.* Beverly Hills, CA: Sage.

Methodological Designs

Blank, D. M. (1985). Development of the Infant Tenderness Scale. *Nursing Research, 34*(4), 211-216.

Manfredi, C. (1986). Reliability and validity of the Phaneuf Nursing Audit. *Western Journal of Nursing Research, 8*(2), 168-180.

Norbeck, J. S., Lindsey, A. M., & Carrieri, V. L. (1983). Further development of the Norbeck Social Support Questionnaire: Normative data and validity testing. *Nursing Research, 32*(1), 4-9.

Toth, J. C. (1986). The Basic Knowledge Assessment Tool (BKAT)—Validity and reliability: A national study of critical care nursing knowledge. *Western Journal of Nursing Research, 8*(2), 181-196.

Name Index

Subject Index

About the Authors

Pamela J. Brink, R.N., FAAN, received her B.S. from Mount St. Mary's College in Los Angeles, her M.S.N. in psychiatric nursing from Catholic University, and her Ph.D. in cultural anthropology from Boston University. She has published two books (*Transcultural Nursing*, 1976; *Basic Steps in Planning Nursing Research*, 1978, 1982, 1988, with Marilynn J. Wood) and numerous articles and book chapters, and is the Founder and Executive Editor of the *Western Journal of Nursing Research*. She is currently Professor and Associate Dean, Research, in the Faculty of Nursing, University of Alberta, Edmonton, Alberta, Canada.

Kathleen C. Buckwalter, Ph.D., R.N., is an Associate Professor at the University of Iowa College of Nursing. Following postdoctoral studies in geriatric mental health, her clinical and research interests have included the development, implementation, and evaluation of innovative geropsychiatric service delivery programs, especially those targeted for the mentally ill elderly in rural environments.

Laurie K. Glass is Associate Professor and Director of the Historical Gallery at the University of Wisconsin—Milwaukee School of Nursing. She received her Ph.D. in nursing research and nursing history from the University of Illinois at Chicago in 1983. Her specific interest is the historical analysis of nursing leaders and their impact on issues and events. She is a member of various national committees that focus on nursing history, and is a past-president of the Wisconsin Nurses Association. She also is an Adjunct Associate Professor at the University of Illinois at Chicago College of Nursing.

317

Nancy R. Lackey is Associate Professor of Nursing at the University of Kansas School of Nursing. She holds a B.S.N. from Indiana University, an M.S.N. from Marquette University, and a Ph.D. in nursing from Texas Woman's University. Her primary interest has been in theory development and validation of the defining characteristics of nursing diagnoses. Her current research focuses on noninstitutionalized cancer patients and their primary caregivers.

Meridean L. Maas, Ph.D., R.N., is an Assistant Professor at the University of Iowa College of Nursing. Her clinical and research interests include nursing diagnosis and interventions for the institutionalized elderly and the design of organizational structures that facilitate professional nursing practice.

Janet C. Meininger is an Associate Professor of Nursing and Epidemiology at the University of Texas Health Science Center at Houston. She received her B.S.N. from St. Louis University, her M.S.N. from Case Western Reserve University with a clinical specialty in public health nursing, and her Ph.D. in epidemiology from the University of North Carolina, Chapel Hill. Her interests include cardiovascular risk factors in children, behavioral factors, health services research, and family health. She has published research papers on these topics as well as articles on research methodology in journals such as *Nursing Research, Journal of Chronic Diseases,* and *Social Science and Medicine.*

Merle H. Mishel is Professor of Nursing at the University of Arizona. She holds a Ph.D. in social psychology from Claremont Graduate School and has authored several papers in the area of instrument development and testing that have appeared in several scholarly nursing research journals. Her interests include the development of instruments to index nursing concepts and the development of the theory of uncertainty in illness. She is currently conducting research in the areas of quality of life following heart transplantation and bereavement resolution.

Patricia L. Munhall, R.N., Ed.D., is a Professor in the Graduate Program of Nursing at Hunter College of the City University of New York. She has published and presented papers extensively on qualitative research. She is coeditor with Carolyn J. Oiler, of the A.J.N. Award-winning textbook *Nursing Research: A Qualitative Perspective*.

Anita L. Wingate is an Associate Professor in the Department of Medical-Surgical Nursing in the School of Nursing, University of Kansas Medical Center. She holds a B.S.N. in nursing and a Ph.D. in anatomy, both from the University of Kansas. Her major teaching and research interests have been in oncology nursing.

Marilynn J. Wood is Dean of Faculty of Nursing at the University of Alberta. Her doctorate is from the School of Public Health at UCLA, in gerontology and biostatistics. She is coauthor of a basic nursing research text and was recipient of an American Journal of Nursing Book of the Year Award in 1984. Her current research is in the area of lifestyle changes related to the treatment of obesity. She is Associate Editor of the *Western Journal of Nursing Research*.

Level	Design Level	Design
III	experimental	experimental
		quasi-experimental
II	survey	comparative
		correlational
I	exploratory-descriptive	descriptive
		exploratory